Glaucoma Surgery

Atlas

Glaucoma Surgery

Atlas

Stephen A. Obstbaum, MD
Director of Ophthalmology
Lenox Hill Hospital

Professor of Clinical Ophthalmology
Cornell University Medical Center
New York, New York

Illustrated by
Sam Potthoff

APPLETON & LANGE
Norwalk, Connecticut/San Mateo, California

0-8385-3270-5

Notice: Our knowledge in clinical sciences is constantly changing. As new information becomes available, changes in treatment and in the use of drugs become necessary. The authors and the publisher of this volume have taken care to make certain that the doses of drugs and schedules of treatment are correct and compatible with the standards generally accepted at the time of publication. The reader is advised to consult carefully the instruction and information material included in the package insert of each drug or therapeutic agent before administration. This advice is especially important when using new or infrequently used drugs.

91 92 93 94 95/ 10 9 8 7 6 5 4 3 2 1

Prentice Hall International (UK) Limited, *London*
Prentice Hall of Australia Pty. Limited, *Sydney*
Prentice Hall Canada, Inc., *Toronto*
Prentice Hall Hispanoamericana, S.A., *Mexico*
Prentice Hall of India Private Limited, *New Delhi*
Prentice Hall of Japan, Inc., *Tokyo*
Simon & Schuster Asia Pte. Ltd., *Singapore*
Editora Prentice Hall do Brasil Ltda., *Rio de Janeiro*
Prentice Hall, *Englewood Cliffs, New Jersey*

Library of Congress Cataloging-in-Publication Data

Obstbaum, Stephen A.
Glaucoma surgery atlas / Stephen A. Obstbaum.
p. cm.
Includes bibliographical references.
Includes index.
ISBN 0-8385-3270-5
1. Glaucoma—Surgery—Atlases. I. Title.
[DNLM: 1. Glaucoma—surgery—atlases. WW 17 014g]
RE871.026 1991
617.7'41059—dc20
DNLM/DLC 90-14513
for Library of Congress CIP

Acquisitions Editor: Joan T. Meyer
Production Editor: Elizabeth C. Ryan
Designer: Steven M. Byrum

ISBN 0-8385-3270-5
90000>
9 780838 532706

PRINTED IN THE UNITED STATES OF AMERICA

To Merilee, Jesse, Lauren, and Jamie for your loving support

Contributors

Kenneth R. Barasch, MD
Assistant Clinical Professor of Ophthalmology
Department of Ophthalmology
Mount Sinai School of Medicine

Lenox Hill Hospital
New York, New York

Carl B. Camras, MD
Associate Professor of Ophthalmology
Department of Ophthalmology
Mount Sinai School of Medicine
New York, New York

Theodore Krupin, MD
Professor of Ophthalmology
Department of Ophthalmology
Northwestern University Medical School
Chicago, Illinois

Steven M. Podos, MD
Professor and Chairman
Department of Ophthalmology
Mount Sinai School of Medicine
New York, New York

Contents

Preface

This atlas presents an approach to the variety of surgical procedures performed in the eye with glaucoma. Our purpose is to describe and illustrate the technical steps of each procedure that have given long-term success. We freely acknowledge that alternative surgical methods exist that might be equally successful. While there are nuances in all forms of surgical intervention, certain basic principles, when judiciously applied, provide consistently satisfactory results. Dynamic developments in ophthalmology impact on the methods used to treat glaucoma. The surgical spectrum of laser treatment to implantation of setons for failed cases and in those with neovascularization reflect these relatively recent developments. The contents of this atlas endeavor to present a reasoned approach to the elements of glaucoma surgery. It is clearly not an end unto itself, but a link in our progress toward improved surgical outcome.

Stephen A. Obstbaum, MD

Glaucoma Surgery

Atlas

1

Anatomy

The success of surgical treatment for glaucoma depends on several factors. These include (1) an understanding of the underlying pathophysiology of the condition producing increased pressure, (2) knowledge of the anatomic landmarks requisite for the particular procedure, (3) performing the procedure as atraumatically as possible, and (4) the individual healing response of the patient. The surgeon is capable of influencing the first three of these factors. Although success in glaucoma surgery is not necessarily assured even with the most skillfully performed procedure, adhering to the principles of surgical technique positively influences a favorable outcome. Comfort with anatomic landmarks is an important ingredient in the surgical approach to the particular glaucomatous state.

ANGLE ANATOMY

Our evaluation of the anterior chamber angle anatomy distinguishes the type of primary glaucoma, assesses degrees of angle width, identifies pigmentary and inflammatory cells, and is crucial for the correct application of laser energy to angle structures.

Schwalbe's line is the end of Descemet's membrane and the anterior extension of the trabecular meshwork. It appears as a slightly raised ridge gonioscopically.

The trabecular meshwork has a uveal and a corneoscleral component. The internal trabecular fibers form the uveal meshwork, whereas the deepest fibers that originate at the corneoscleral junction extend posteriorly to insert at the scleral spur.

The scleral spur marks the innermost anterior extension of the sclera and is the area to which the ciliary body attaches, as well as to the fibers of the corneoscleral trabeculum. It appears as a grayish line just anterior to the angle recess.

Schlemm's canal lies just behind the trabecular meshwork. Often, blood in Schlemm's canal makes this structure more visible. Under this circumstance, it is seen anterior to the scleral spur.

The ciliary muscle inserts into the scleral spur and forms the angle recess along with a peripheral portion of the iris.

Figure 1–1. Most glaucoma filtering surgery is performed in the region of the corneoscleral limbus. When the conjunctiva and Tenon's layers have been removed, either by a limbal or a fornix-based flap, we can visualize the anatomy of this area. Most conspicuous is the demarcation between the scleral fibers and the blue-gray zone anterior to it and extending forward to the corneal tissue. The alteration in color of the limbal region occurs because of an interdigitation of the corneal fibers into the scleral tissue. One can think of a somewhat triangular wedge of corneal tissue with its apex pointed posteriorly, invested by two wedges of scleral tissue with their apices facing anteriorly. This tissue area is neither totally corneal nor is it scleral, thus causing a variation in color.

The posterior, or scleral, border of the limbus is 0–1.5 mm from the point of reflection of the conjunctival–corneal junction at Bowman's membrane. The internal structure lying perpendicularly beneath this external landmark is within the trabecular meshwork. However, in an eye with a crowded anterior segment, such as one with a short axial length and angle-closure glaucoma, this incision may pass more posteriorly into the ciliary body. We, therefore, advise making bevelled incisions in this area extending toward the anterior chamber. In this way, adequate entry into the anterior chamber is achieved without the risk of damaging posterior structures and producing uncontrolled bleeding.

The anterior border of the limbus is at the reflection of the conjunctival and corneal epithelia. This area is identified by a prominent bump when the limbal-based conjunctival flap is bluntly reflected forward. This is an important landmark in performing the trabecular surgery, to be discussed later, because, once this area is delineated, adequate lamellar dissection slightly anterior to this point permits excision of a deep scleral block of tissue that will include some peripheral cornea as well as the trabeculum. An incision made perpendicularly in this area will enter the chamber at or slightly anterior to Schwalbe's line.

Since most filtering procedures are performed at the superior limbus, the width of the limbus is fairly uniform through the upper 90 degrees. However, the external landmarks of the limbus become narrower as the nasal and temporal aspects of the limbus are approached. If secondary procedures are performed in these areas, this fact should be borne in mind so that appropriate adjustments in technique are observed.

Identification of Schlemm's canal is required in the trabeculotomy procedure. It is difficult to localize this structure without a good knowledge of the normal anatomy. If one remembers that the scleral posterior border of the limbus overlies the scleral spur and that Schlemm's canal generally is just anterior to this structure, adequate localization is possible.

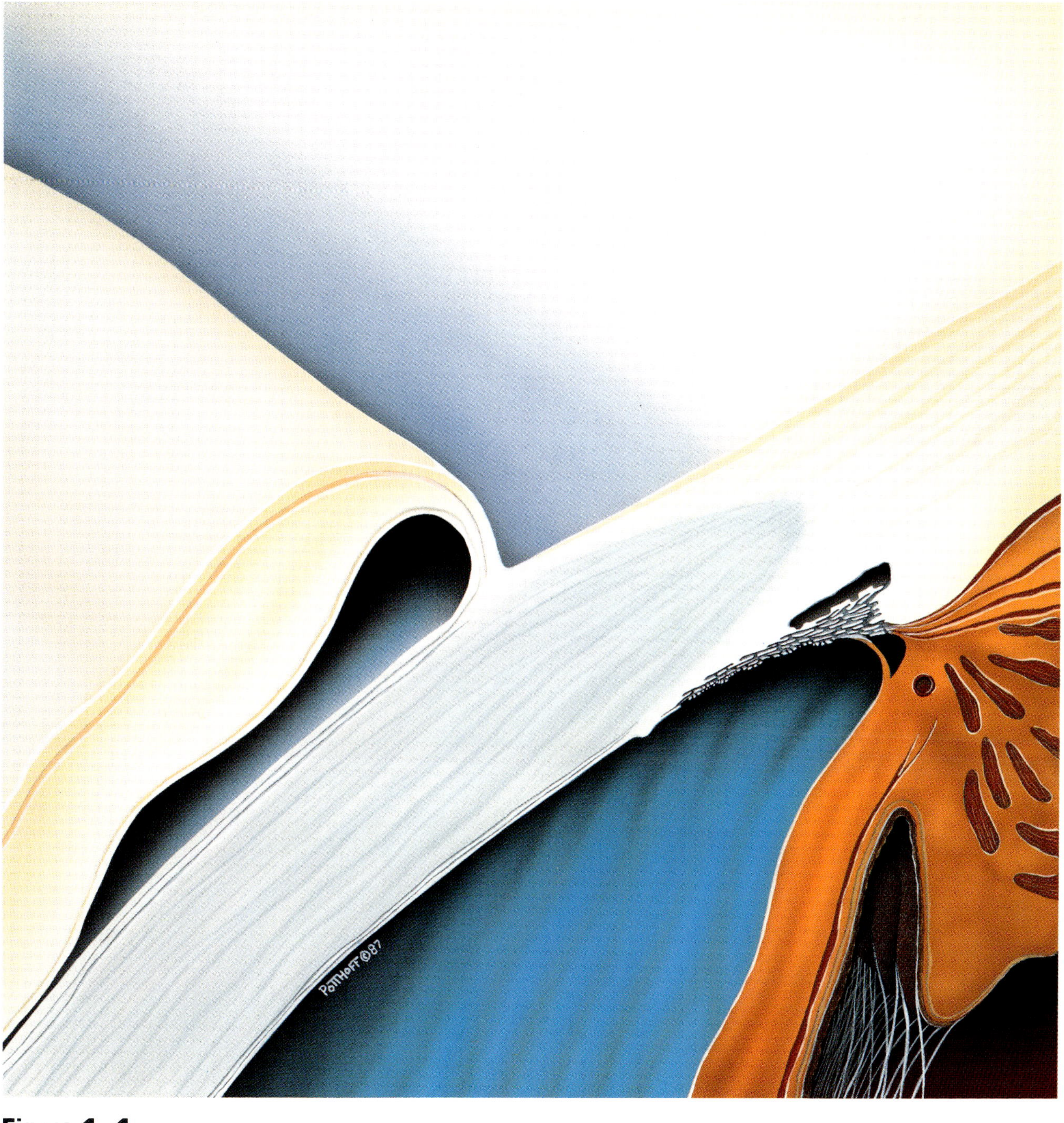

Figure 1–1

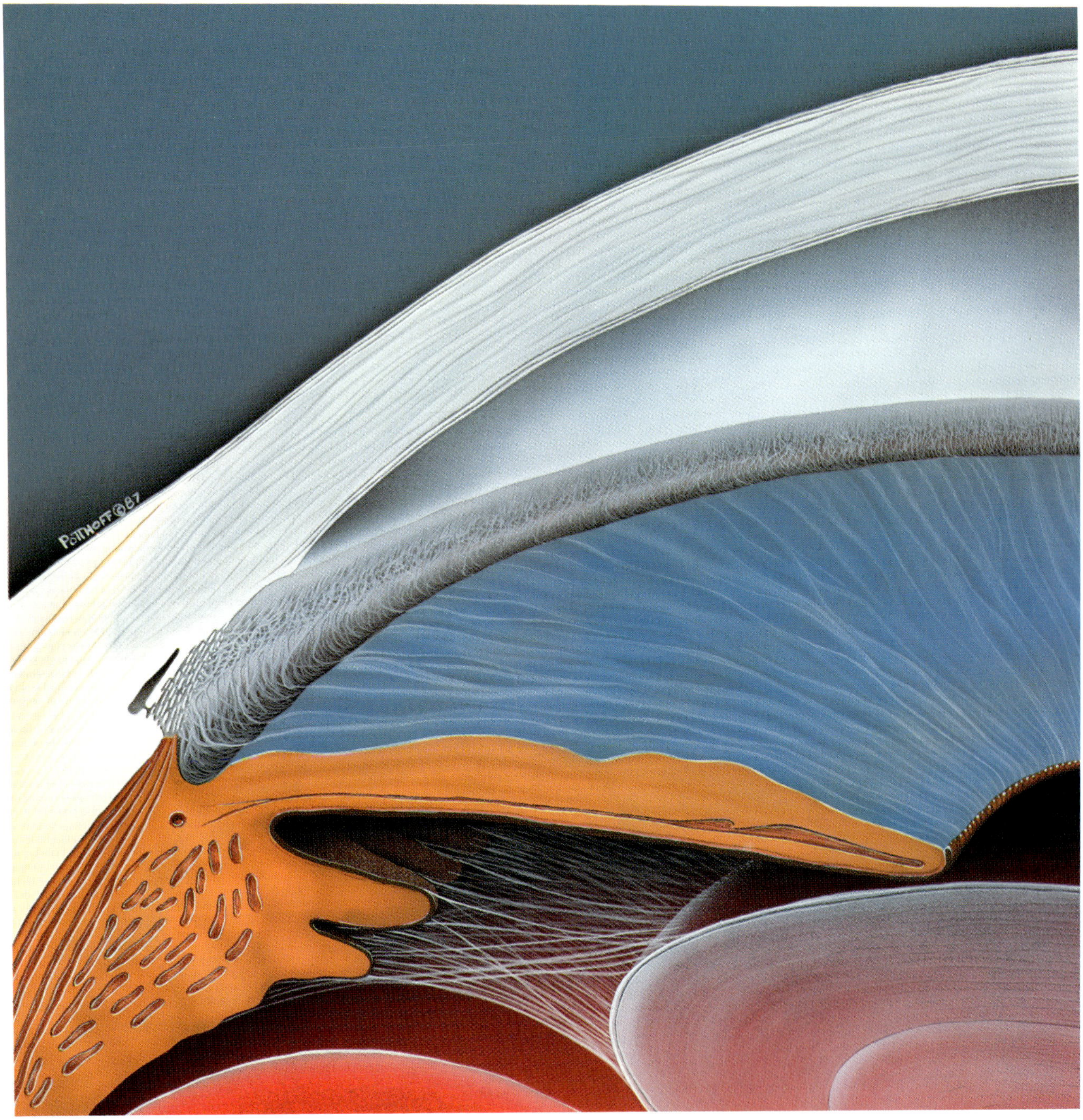

Figure 1–2

Figure 1–2. The iris root lies just anterior to the scleral spur. It is, therefore, beneath the posterior limbal border and approximately 1.5–2.0 mm from the anterior demarcation of the limbus. If one performs a peripheral iridectomy through an ad externo procedure under a conjunctival flap, an incision that is too perpendicular may enter the ciliary body, whereas one that is too bevelled might result in an iridectomy that is not adequately basal.

The iris is composed of two layers: a stromal layer and a pigmented layer. In performing a surgical iridectomy, it is important to be assured that both layers of the iris have been excised so that a patent opening is achieved. Similarly, vagaries in the color of the iris will influence the success of argon laser iridectomy in developing a through-and-through opening. With the neodymium:YAG (Nd:YAG) laser, iris color is not as important.

The ciliary body is anchored at the scleral spur anteriorly and extends posteriorly as the pars plicata and the pars plana. The former structure is about 3 mm in extent from the scleral spur. When cyclodestructive procedures are performed, the applications are placed in the region to influence the ciliary processes to secrete aqueous humor. The pars plana is behind the pars plicata and extends about 4 mm posteriorly. This is a region through which access to the vitreous cavity is attained. Posterior sclerotomies are made somewhere between 3.5 and 5.0 mm from the anterior limit of the limbus.

Major vessels to the anterior segment of the eye follow the course of the horizontal and vertical rectus muscles. These anterior ciliary arteries should be avoided when incisions are made through the superficial tissues of the eye, especially when entering the suprachoroidal space in the cyclodialysis procedure. It is wisest to enter the quadrants between the rectus muscles.

2

Mechanisms of Angle-Closure Glaucoma

The clinical characteristic of angle-closure glaucoma is the obstruction of the anterior chamber angle by iris tissue, resulting in a reduction of aqueous outflow and an elevated intraocular pressure. There are four major mechanisms of angle-closure glaucoma: (1) pupillary block, (2) ciliary block (malignant glaucoma), (3) creeping angle closure, and (4) plateau iris.

Figure 2–1. The pupillary block mechanism is the most frequently encountered. In this condition, several physiologic events combine to produce the classic picture. Usually, the eye is hyperopic and has a short axial length with a shallow anterior chamber. The crystalline lens is anteriorly situated and shifts farther forward as the zonules become lax. When the pupil is in a middilated position, a blockage occurs between the anteriorly situated lens and the iris that reduces aqueous flow into the anterior chamber. The aqueous accumulates behind the iris, billowing the flaccid peripheral iris forward to obstruct the filtration angle. Peripheral anterior synechia formation resulting in permanent areas of angle-closure glaucoma may occur with repeated subacute attacks or when inflammation ensues.

Figure 2–2. Ciliary block (ciliolenticular block, ciliovitreal block) also has been termed "malignant glaucoma." This entity was described initially as occurring after successful surgery for acute angle-closure glaucoma. However, there is a variety of conditions that also may lead to posterior pooling of aqueous humor either within or behind the vitreous body. The misdirected aqueous alters the anatomic relationships anterior to it, so that contact between these structures prevents the forward flow of aqueous. Not infrequently, the ciliary processes are noted to touch the lens and even to rotate anteriorly. As in pupillary block, the laxity of the zonules causes anterior positioning of the lens.

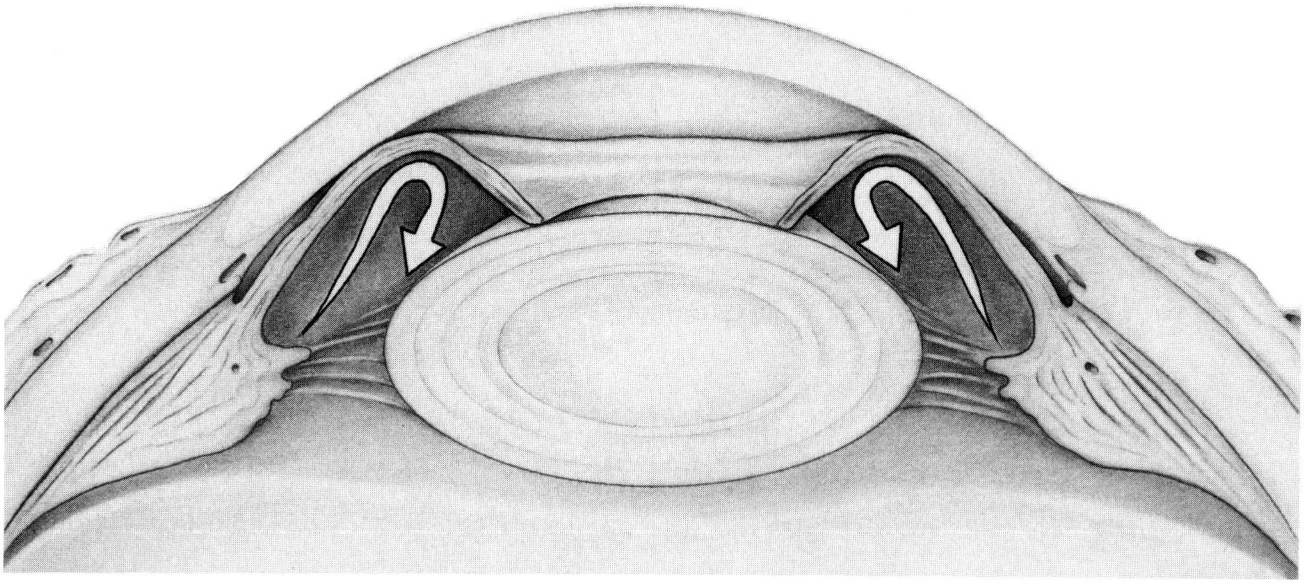

Figure 2–1

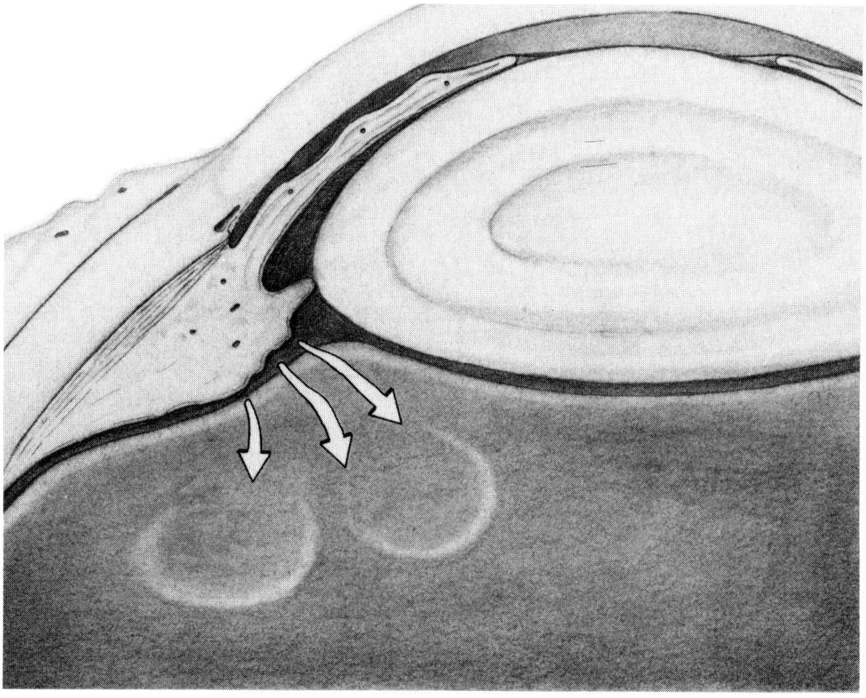

Figure 2–2

Figure 2–3A, B, and C. Creeping angle closure is characterized by synechial closure of the angle recess from a posterior to an anterior position. This is a progressive process (note A to B to C) that eventuates in obstruction from the depth of the angle to a point anterior to the trabecular meshwork. This form of angle-closure glaucoma can produce chronic angle closure that frequently mimics open-angle glaucoma in the profundity of visual field loss and optic nerve changes.

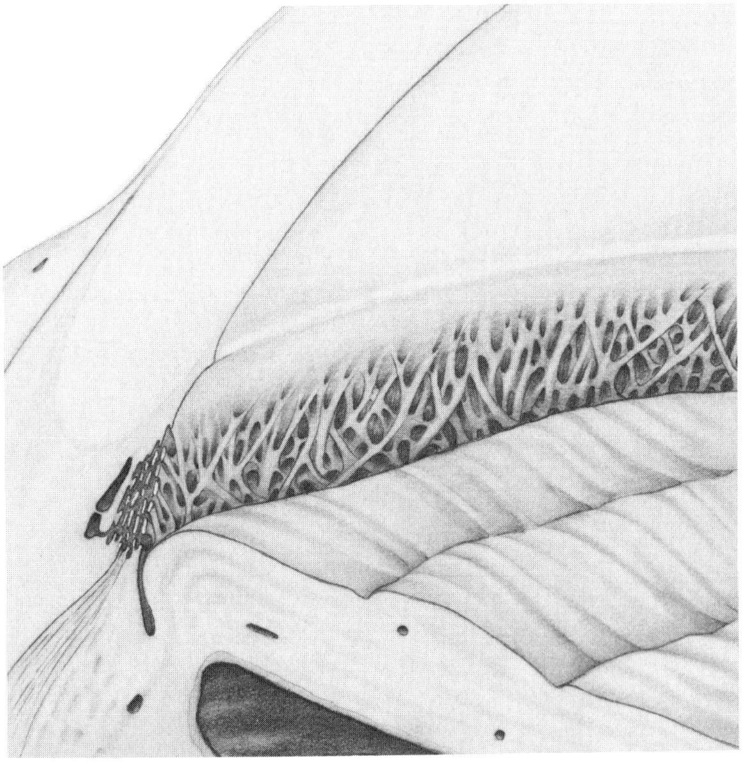

Figure 2–3A

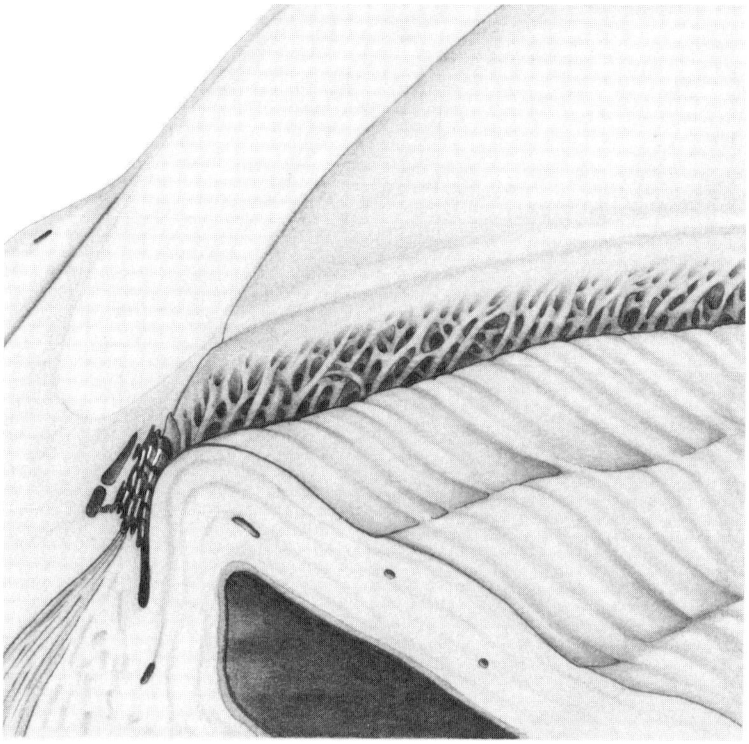

Figure 2–3B

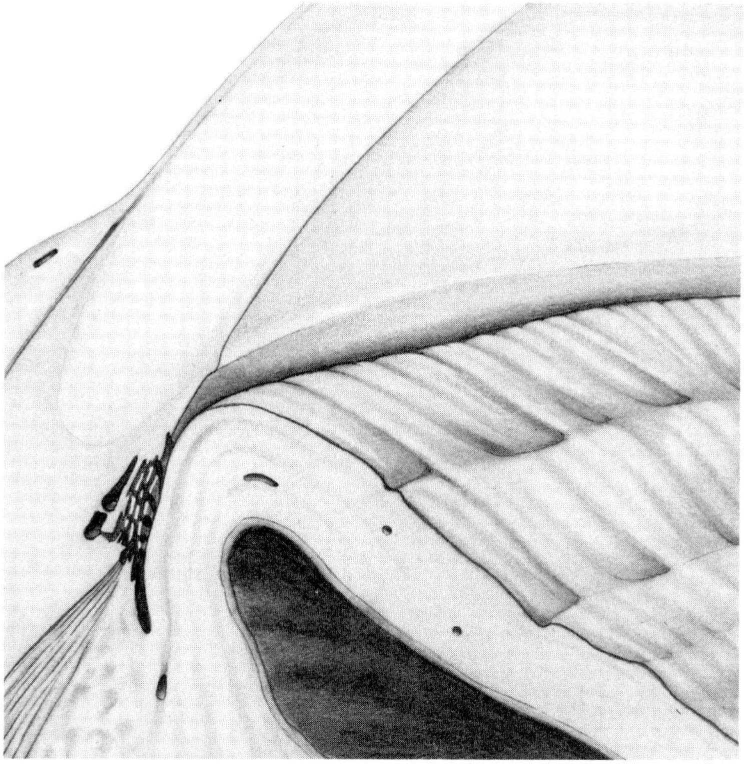

Figure 2–3C

Figure 2–4. Plateau iris angle closure occurs in eyes that have a flat anterior insertion of the iris on the ciliary body. Pupil dilation produces peripheral corrugation of the iris that obstructs the aqueous outflow through the trabecular meshwork. Since the presentation of angle-closure glaucoma can be varied, recognition of the mechanisms involved will permit the application of a rational approach to treating these cases.

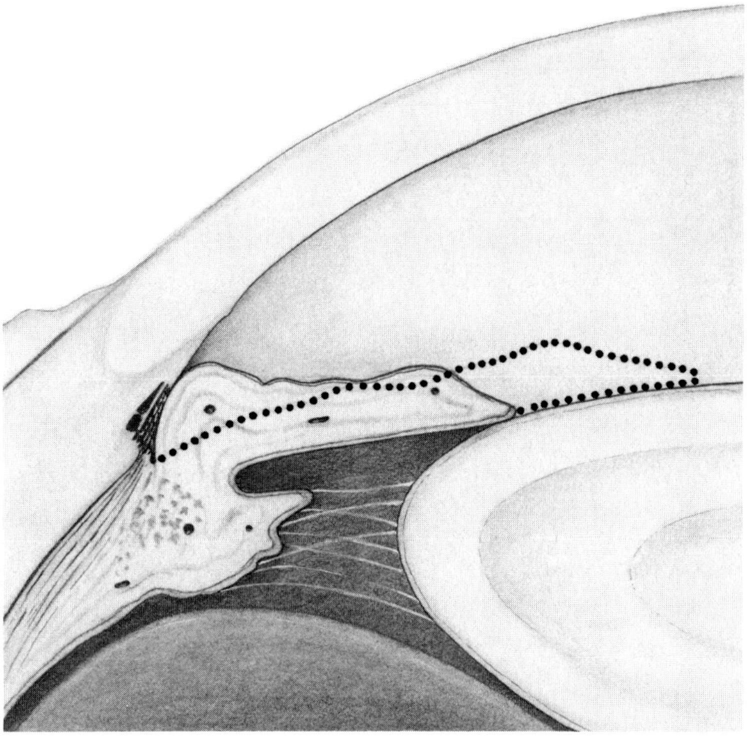

Figure 2–4

3

Laser Iridectomy

The use of laser energy to create a through-and-through opening in the iris has, for the most part, obviated the need for primary surgical iridectomy. This latter procedure is the classic treatment for angle-closure glaucoma, since it creates a communication between the posterior and anterior chambers, bypassing dependence on the pupillary flow of aqueous. The argon and neodymium:YAG (Nd:YAG) lasers are capable also of producing an iris opening that shunts posteriorly produced aqueous through to the anterior chamber and breaks the sequence of pupillary block. Since the eye is not entered, use of the argon and Nd:YAG lasers is favored at present.

GENERAL CONSIDERATIONS

Several drops of a miotic agent, such as 2% pilocarpine, are instilled to make the pupil miotic and place the iris on stretch. During an attack of angle-closure glaucoma, the cornea is hazy, the anterior chamber is shallow, and the pupil is mid-dilated. Osmotic agents should be administered systemically to reduce vitreous volume, reduce intraocular pressure (IOP) and the consequent iris ischemia, and permit the miotic agent to exert its effect on the pupil. The chamber will deepen and the cornea will clear somewhat with reduction of IOP.

Figure 3–1. With the pupil in a miotic state, topical anesthetic drops are applied to the cornea, and an Abraham contact lens is inserted between the lids. The Abraham lens with a +66-diopter inset segment concentrates the energy and focuses the power of the laser source. In addition, it separates the lids and allows the surgeon to steady the globe during the procedure.

Figure 3–2. The upper quadrants between 9 and 11 o'clock, and 1 and 3 o'clock are preferred areas to perform the laser iridectomy, although an alternative site can be selected. Among the advantages of performing the iridectomy more superiorly are that the effect of induced polycoria is clinically less significant in this area, and the gas bubbles, which are often generated during laser iridectomy and which move superiorly in the chamber, do not obscure the surgeon's view.

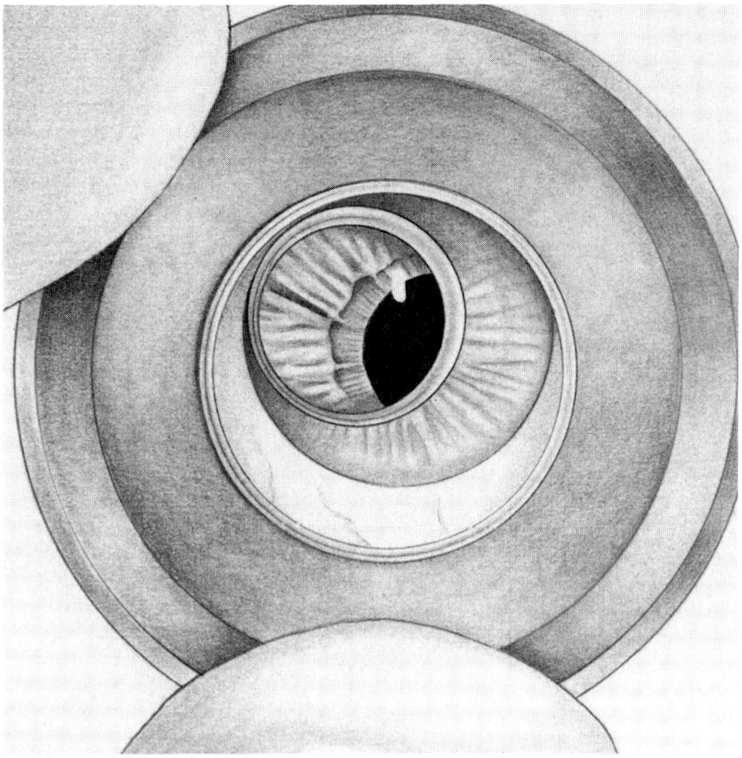

Figure 3–1

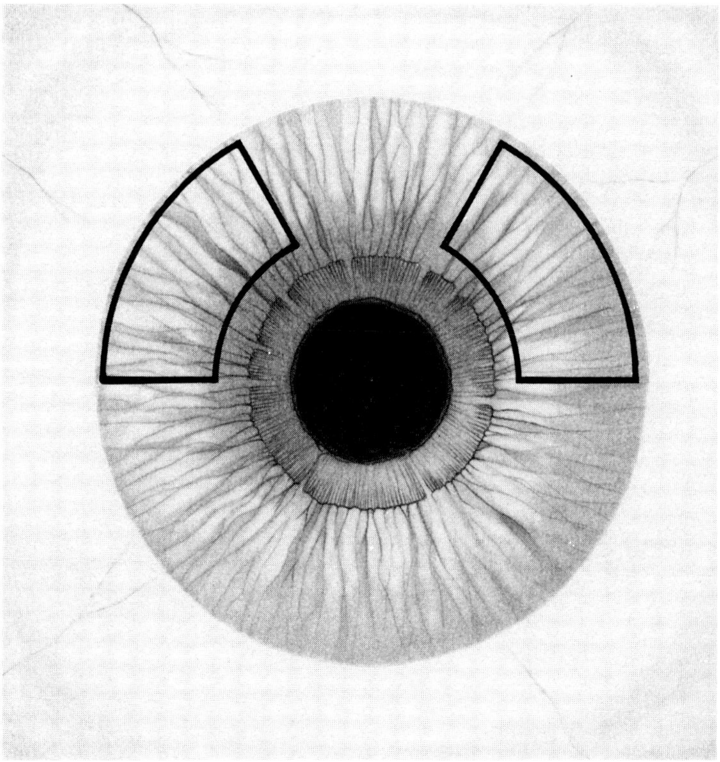

Figure 3–2

Figure 3–3. It is advantageous to deliver laser energy through a relatively thinned portion of the iris. An iris crypt located within the areas we have designated in Figure 3–2 is selected. The laser iridectomy should be situated one half to two thirds the distance from the pupillary sphincter to the peripheral portion of the iris. Although in classic surgical iridectomy, the teaching is to clear the periphery of the lens, placing the laser iridectomy in the position described does not promote obstruction of the opening.

Figure 3–4. A circle of low-energy burns produces a drumhead configuration of the iris tissue contained within the encircling burns. In effect, this thins the tissue by pulling it taut to permit easier penetration in the central area. This technique can be performed also with light brown or medium brown irides when an iris crypt is not evident in the area designated for the iridectomy. The settings for these burns are 300 mW, 200 μm spot size, and 0.2-second duration. If an iris crypt is present, this is the desired area for the laser iridectomy. The energy should be delivered to the crypt at its edge overlapping an iris pillar, since the iridectomy will widen to a greater extent than if the depth of the crypt is chosen.

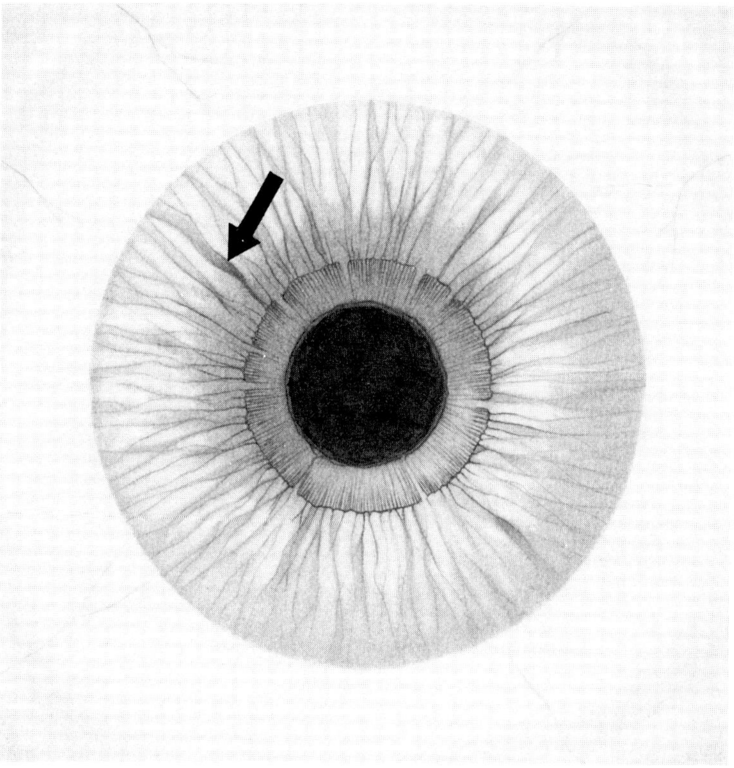

Figure 3–3

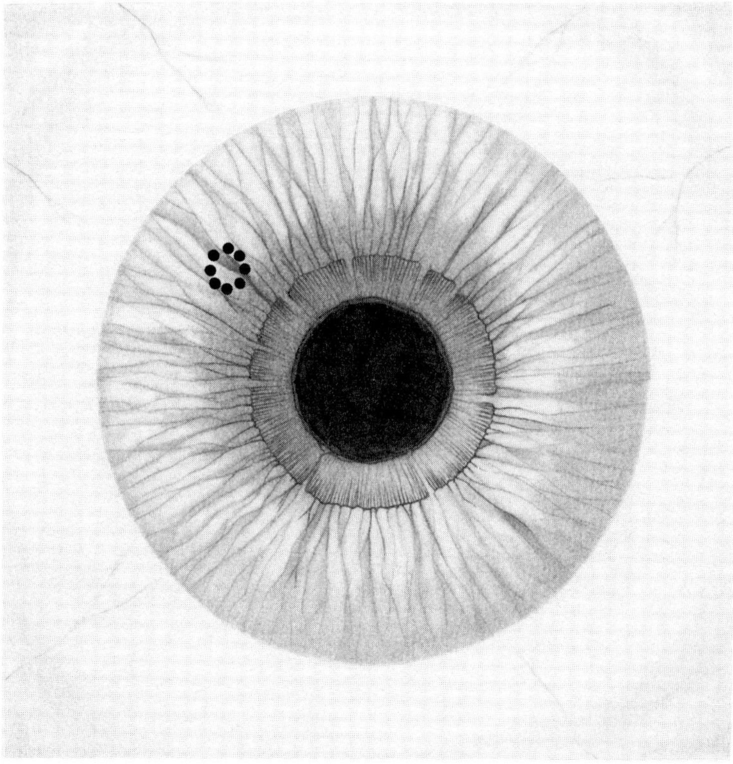

Figure 3–4

Figure 3–5. This cross-sectional representation shows the effect of the circle of burns on the iris tissues contained within them. The stroma and pigment epithelium are relatively thinned and taut in comparison to the surrounding tissue. In angle-closure glaucoma, where there is some degree of iris bombé and relatively close proximity of the endothelium to the iris, it is advantageous to attempt iris penetration with the lowest amount of energy and the fewest burns.

Figure 3–6. The taut iris in the center of the ring of burns is then penetrated by an argon laser beam directed perpendicular to the surface of the Abraham lens and the plane of the iris. The initial energy settings are typically 1000 mW, 50 μm, 0.2 second. The laser burns are delivered to the iris at the same spot until the stroma is penetrated and the posterior iris pigment layer is reached.

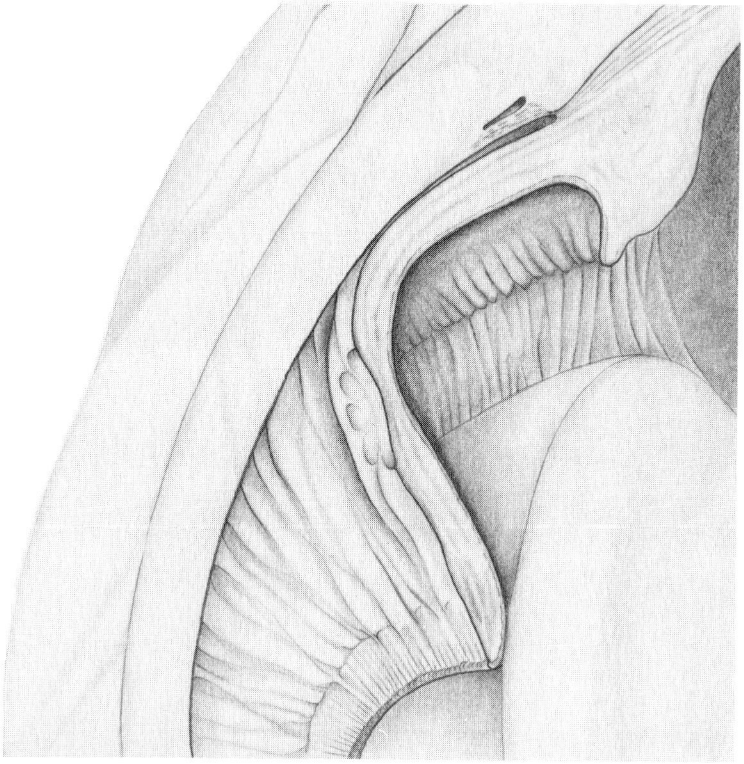

Figure 3–5

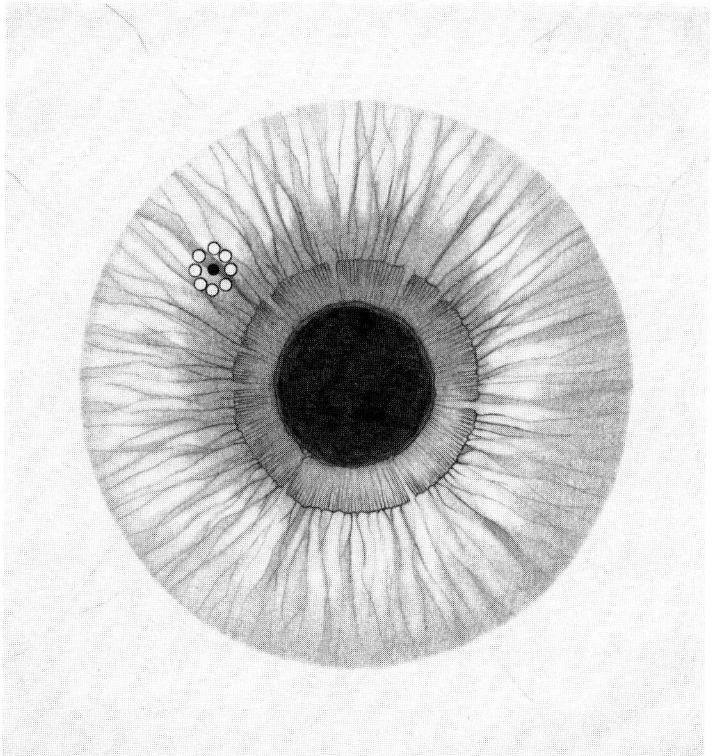

Figure 3–6

Figure 3–7. The cross-sectional view shows penetration in the center of the ring of surrounding burns. The laser beam is delivered perpendicular to the cornea, iris, and contact lens.

Figure 3–8. Once the stromal tissue has been removed, the iris-pigmented epithelium is now visible. Since this layer readily absorbs laser energy and is less dense in its anatomic structure, a puff or mushroom of pigment is released into the aqueous. At this point, the laser energy can be reduced, and cautious laser applications can be applied, directing the laser beam away from the posterior pole.

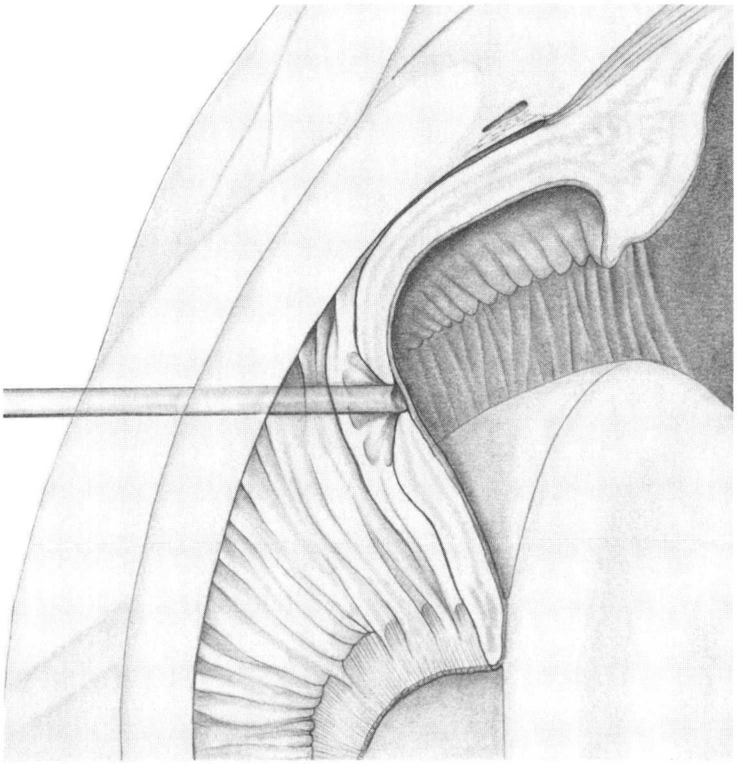

Figure 3–7

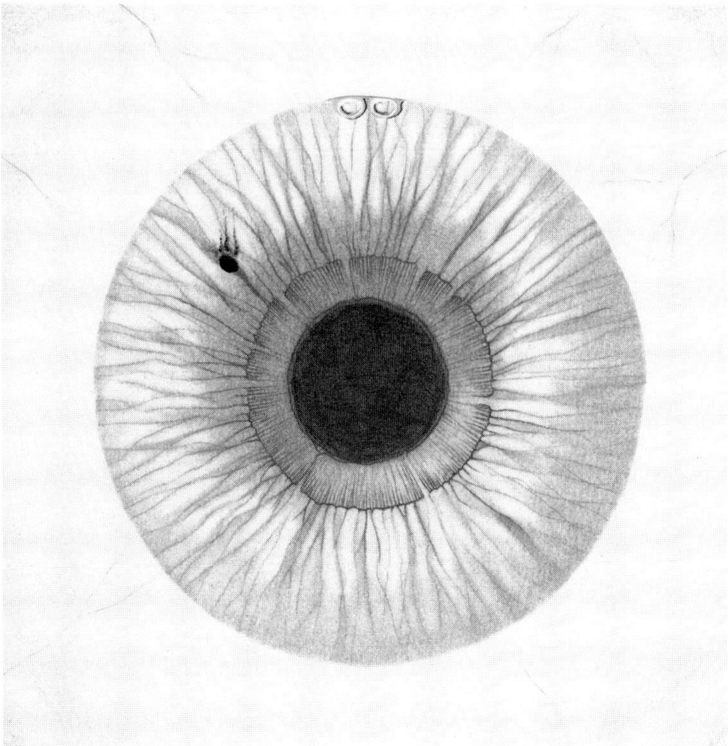

Figure 3–8

Figure 3–9. The end point of a successful laser iridectomy is the appearance of a through-and-through opening and visualization of the anterior lens capsule. Often, a fine, filamentous, gossamer-like layer of the pigment epithelium remains intact at the innermost aspect of the iridectomy site. If the surgeon relies solely on retroillumination to assess the red reflex through the iridectomy, this remaining layer of tissue can be missed. A clear view of the anterior lens capsule beneath the iridectomy is the most desirable end point. Often, the blue-green aiming beam shows fluorescence of the anterior lens capsule.

Figure 3–10. The ease of laser iridectomy is dependent on iris color. Blue and dark brown irides often are resistant to laser penetration. The stroma of blue irides does not absorb the laser energy. The stroma is unaffected, and the energy passes through to the iris pigment epithelium. In effect, the inner portion of the iris tissue (i.e., the pigmented tissue) is removed, whereas the anterior stroma remains intact, thereby preventing a through-and-through opening. With dark brown irides, the converse occurs. Here, the thick stromal tissue absorbs much of the light energy before it can reach the posterior pigmented epithelium. Charring of the stroma occurs, producing a carbonized, shallow crater with inadequate penetration. The method used for the dark brown iris has been termed the "chipping" technique. The laser setting is reduced from 0.2 second to 0.02 second. The spot size remains 50 μm, and the energy delivered can vary from 800 to 1000 mW. The surface of the dark brown iris is chipped away with contiguous burns to make a crater in the stroma that reaches the pigment epithelium. Reducing the exposure time for delivery of the laser burns prevents the dark char that absorbs energy and does not permit penetration. Once the pigment epithelium has been reached, one can increase the time setting to 0.2 second and proceed as with the light brown iris.

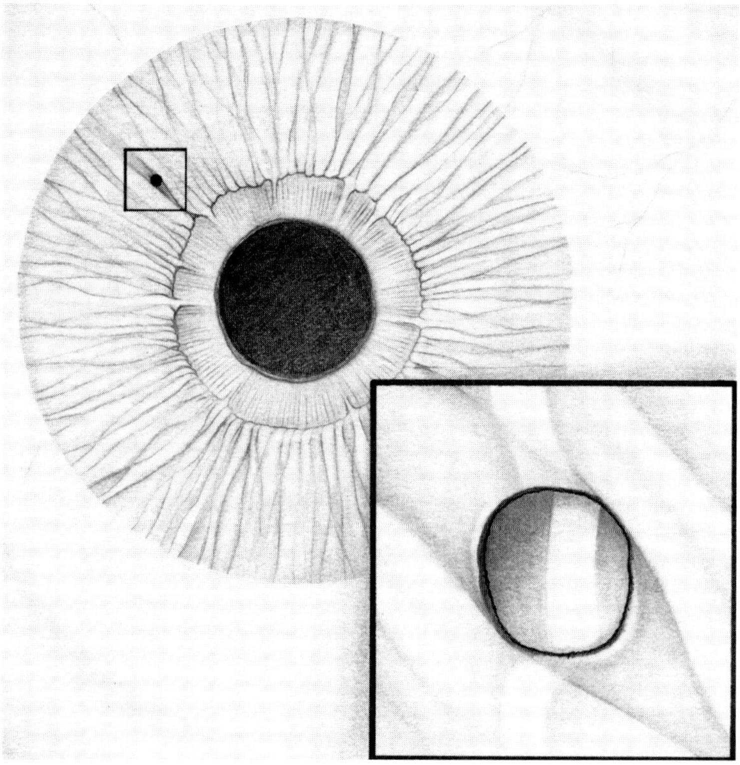

Figure 3–9

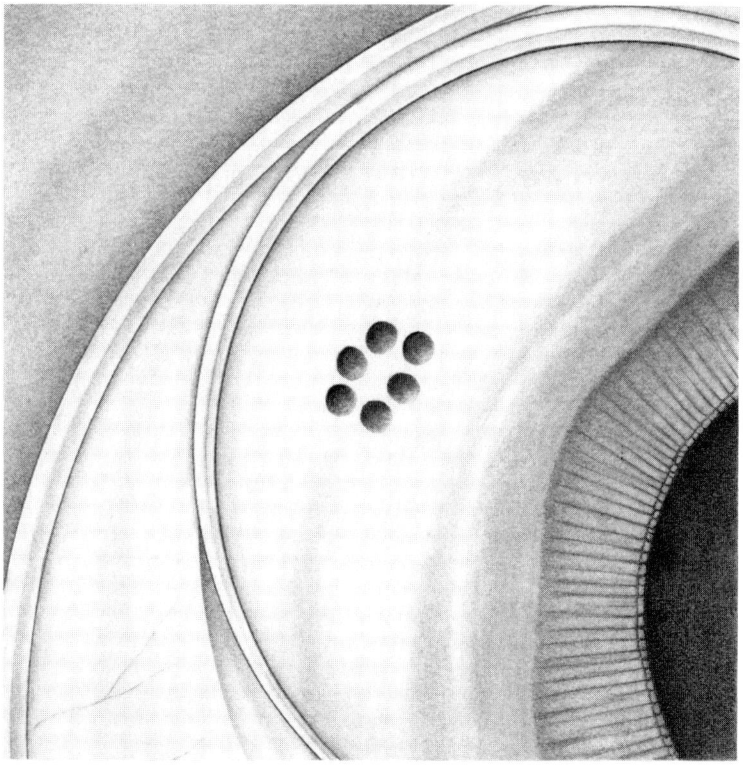

Figure 3–10

Figure 3–11. The other difficult case is the light-colored iris. In this instance, laser energy penetrates the stroma and is absorbed by the pigment epithelium, leaving the overlying stroma intact. The laser settings are changed to increase the power setting to 1500 mW and the time setting to 0.5 second, while keeping the spot sizes at 50 μm. The increased power and time setting permit a slower, more intense burn. The burn generates a gas bubble. As soon as the bubble is noted, pressure on the foot pedal is released and then redepressed to deliver the laser energy while focusing on the air bubble. In this way, the light iris can be penetrated with relatively few applications.

Figure 3–12. The use of the Nd:YAG laser for iris surgery has, for the most part, supplanted the argon laser for iridectomy surgery in my practice. The problem with the light brown and dark blue iris is obviated by this lasing medium. I have used the Abraham lens at a setting of 5 MJ and a single burst. The major difference is that the argon laser coagulates blood vessels, whereas the Nd:YAG laser does not, and, therefore, some bleeding may be encountered. However, gentle pressure on the contact lens often will stem this oozing.

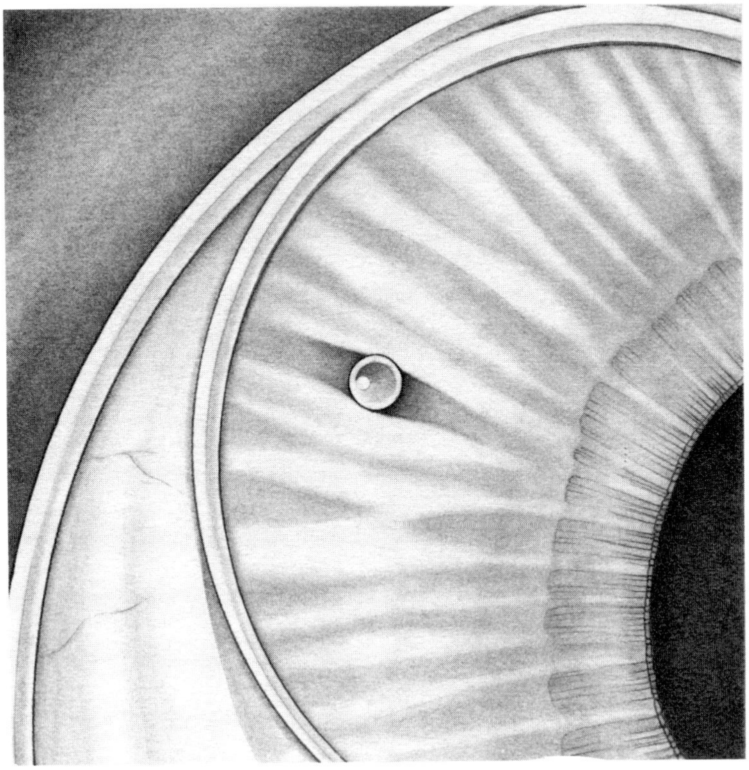

Figure 3–11

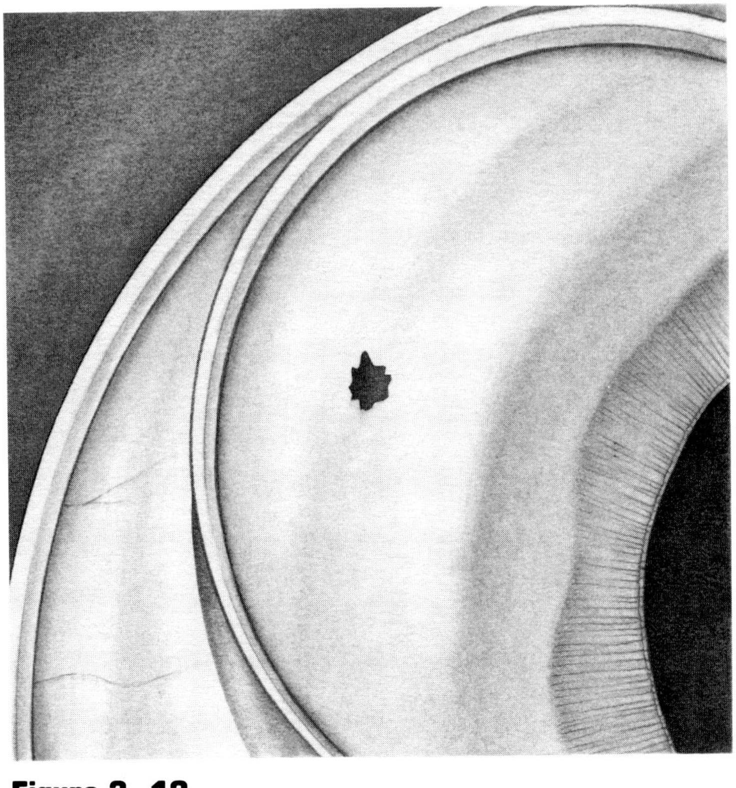

Figure 3–12

Figure 3–13. Gonioplasty or iridoplasty is a technique used to widen the peripheral angle, either as a primary procedure or to prepare the angle for additional therapy. The principle of gonioplasty is to produce low-energy burns to contract the peripheral iris. These burns can be delivered directly through the cornea or indirectly by using a goniolens or Abraham lens.

The settings usually used are a spot size of 200 μm, a power setting 300 mW (greater energy is required if a goniolens is used), and a time of 0.5 second. The most frequent application for gonioplasty is in an eye with open-angle glaucoma requiring laser trabeculoplasty and a narrow angle approach because of iris bombé. Treating the peripheral iris flattens it and widens the angle, which facilitates argon laser treatment. Other uses for this procedure are to break peripheral anterior synechiae, open the angle in neovascular glaucoma, and as a treatment for appositional closure producing angle closure. Another application for gonioplasty is in the treatment of nanophthalmos.

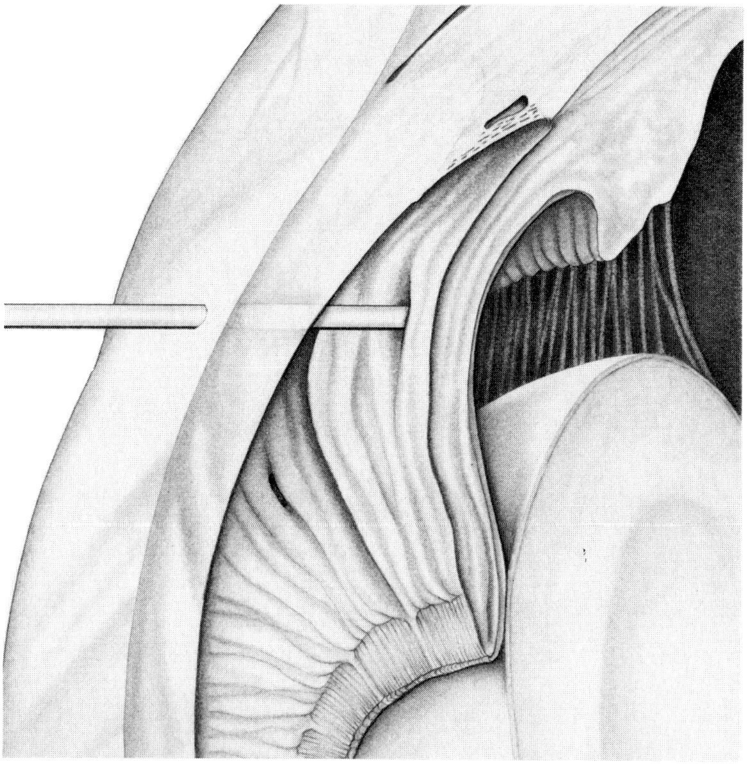

Figure 3–13

4

Surgical Iridectomy

This procedure is the classic surgical treatment for pupillary block angle-closure glaucoma. With the advent of laser treatment, both argon and Nd:YAG, this procedure is performed less frequently than in previous years. There are circumstances, however, in which a surgical iridectomy is required. The operation can be performed ab externo under a conjunctival flap or through a clear corneal incision. We have favored the latter technique because it preserves the conjunctiva and Tenon's tissues should a filtering procedure be required in the future. It is a straightforward method that avoids some of the peculiarities of angle anatomy that may occur in eyes with angle-closure glaucoma.

Figure 4–1. The pupillary block mechanism is characterized by a mid-dilated pupil, iris bombé, shallow anterior chamber and corneal edema. In order to treat this condition, an opening in the iris that obviates aqueous flow through the pupil is desirable.

Figure 4–2. Often, dilating the pupil can break a pupillary block mechanism. However, to treat this condition definitively, either a surgical or laser iridectomy is required. It is undesirable to perform either of these procedures when the pupil is dilated. Therefore, most surgeons do not use dilation to treat pupillary block.

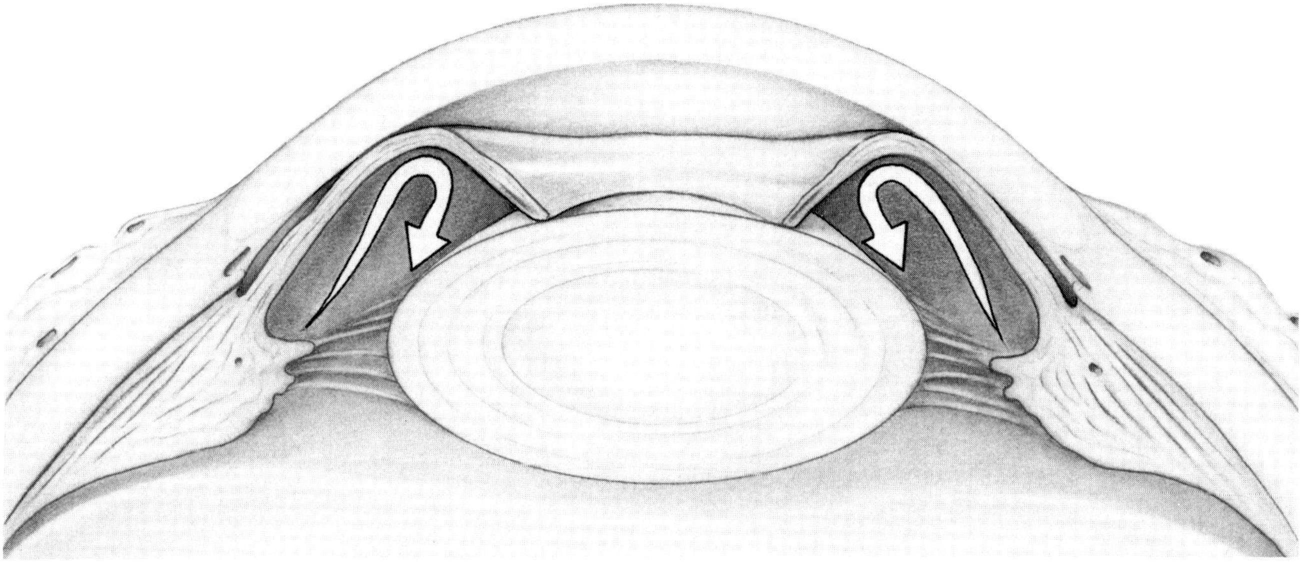

Figure 4–1

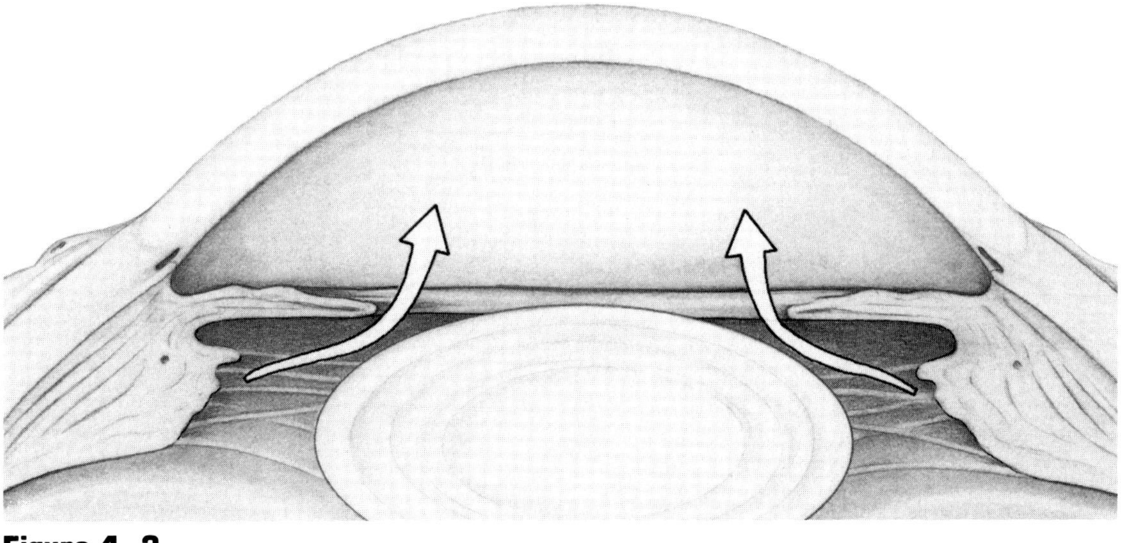

Figure 4–2

Figure 4–3. A cordlike incision is made just within the arcade of superficial corneal vessels. I prefer a site between 10 and 2 o'clock so that the iridectomy will be covered by the upper lid. The superficial incision is made with a rounded blade to the level of Descemet's membrane. It is important to make the incision 2.5–3.0 mm in length, since the deeper portion of the vertical incision generally is not the same length as the external portion. A sharp blade with its cutting edge directed upward then completes the incision into the anterior chamber. A gemstone blade (diamond, sapphire) permits precise control of all aspects of the incision.

Figure 4–4. Gentle pressure applied to the posterior lip of the wound will prolapse iris through the edges of the incision or into the incision per se. If it is at all possible, one should avoid entering the anterior chamber with an instrument to grasp iris tissue, since inadvertent damage to the lens may occur.

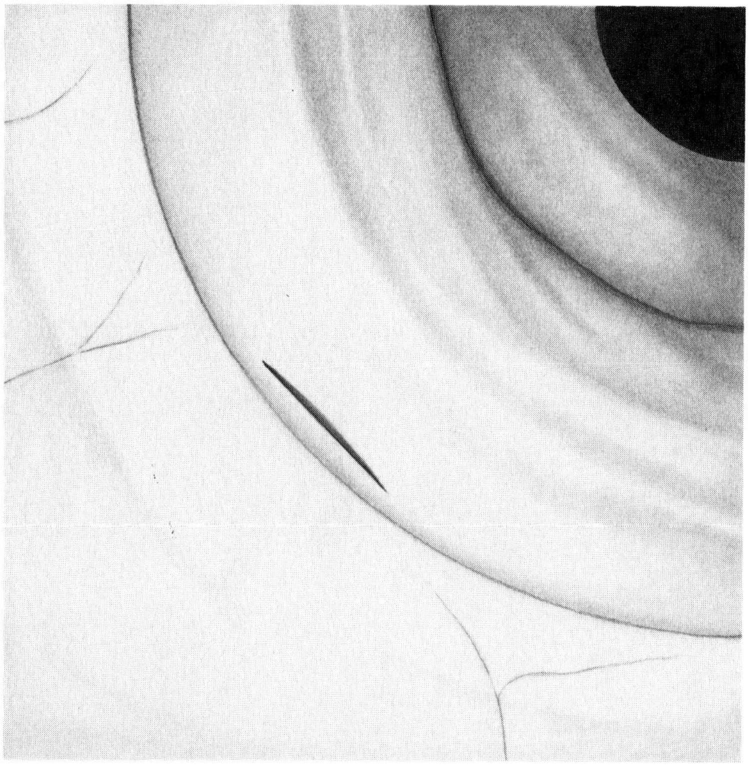

Figure 4–3

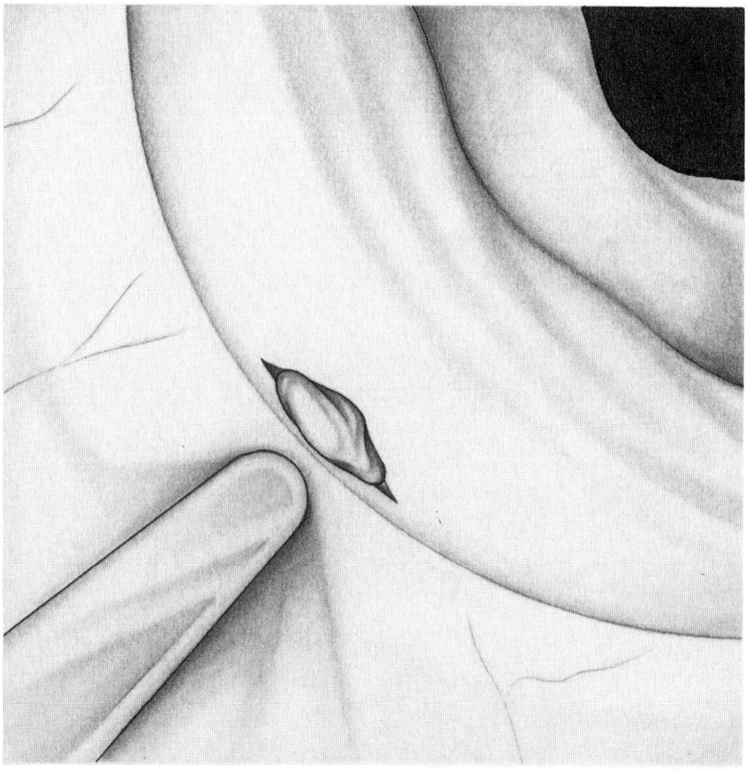

Figure 4–4

Figure 4–5. The iris tissue within the incision is grasped with a toothed forceps. In order to make an adequate peripheral iridectomy that is slightly wider than the incision size, the iris tissue is moved toward the left while an incision is made in its right pillar.

Figure 4–6. The tissue is then moved toward the right, and the left pillar is excised. The iris tissue is inspected, and in addition to stromal tissue, the pigmented epithelial layer should be evident in the specimen. Often, there is residual pigment epithelium or stroma within the edges of the wound. Simply depressing the posterior edge of the incision and gently irrigating, without entering the anterior chamber, will wash the tissue from the incision site and reestablish the correct anatomy.

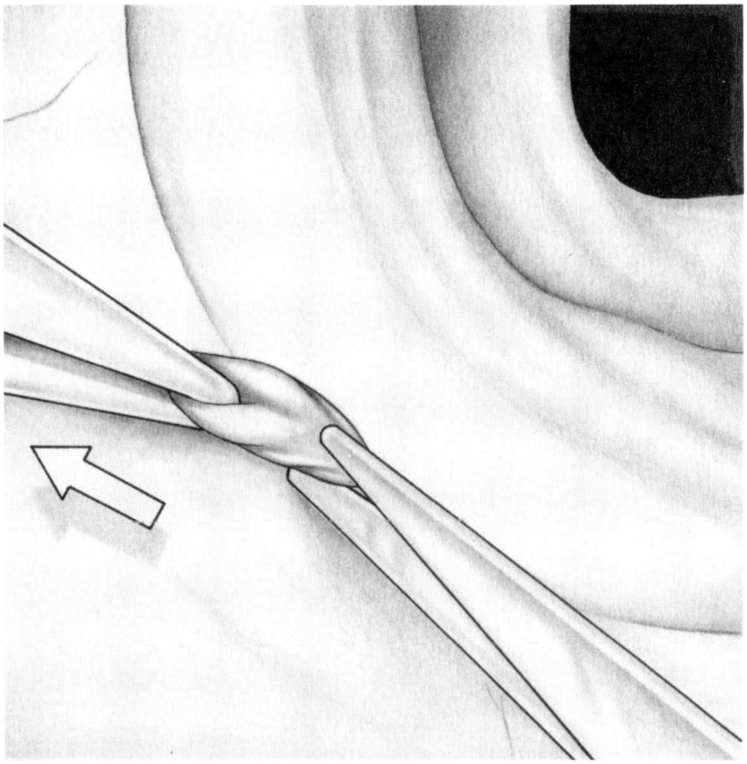

Figure 4–5

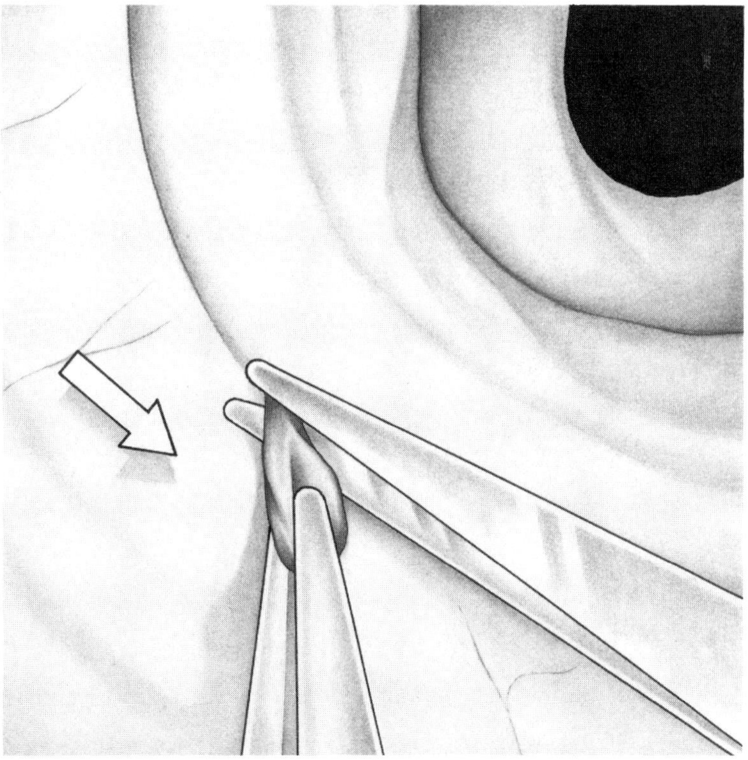

Figure 4–6

Figure 4–7. After the procedure, the iridectomy is complete, and the anterior lens capsule is clearly visualized. The anterior chamber is formed. The incision is closed with a single 10-0 nylon suture. Should the chamber not form after this procedure, a mechanism other than angle-closure should be sought. The most likely mechanism is ciliary-block glaucoma. In the event that iris tissue does not prolapse through the wound edges with pressure on the posterior edge of the incision, it becomes necessary to enter the anterior chamber to exteriorize the iris. It is best, under these circumstances, to use a forceps without teeth to grasp the iris.

Figure 4–8. Often, a toothed forceps will engage only the stroma, leaving the pigment epithelium intact. Consequently, there is no communication between the posterior and anterior chambers, and pupillary block will not be broken. It is wisest not to go after the pigment epithelium directly at this time but rather to treat it with the argon laser, which will create an opening quite easily.

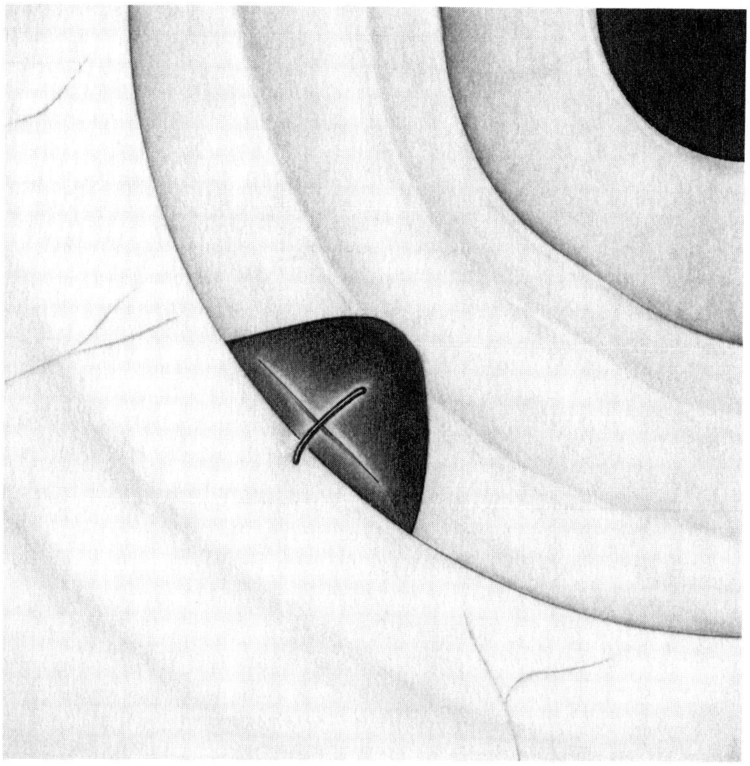

Figure 4–7

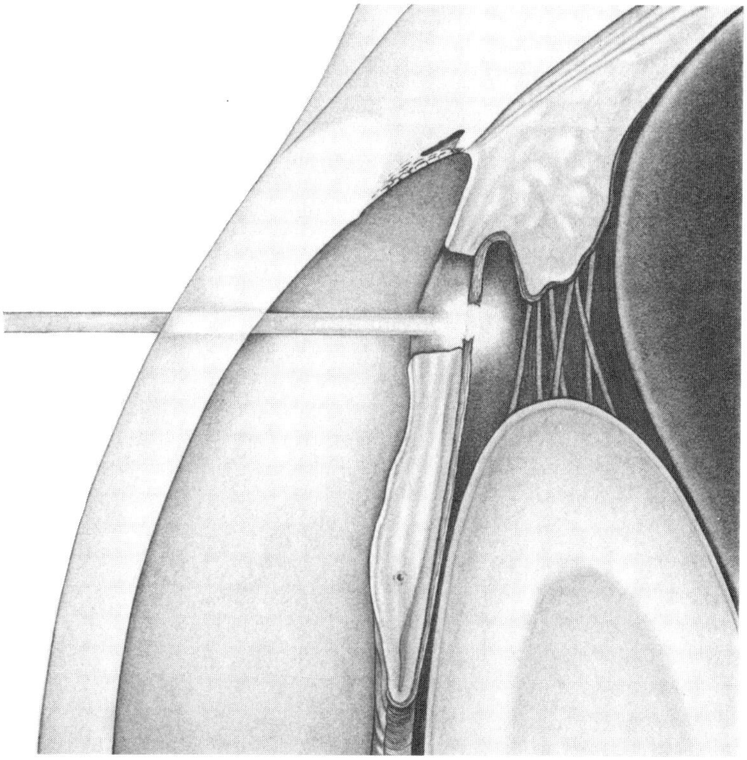

Figure 4–8

Figure 4–9. The need to do a sector iridectomy often arises, either because it is believed that a surgical peripheral iridectomy is inadequate or, more commonly, for optical purposes. Once again, a cordlike incision through clear cornea is made as for the surgical peripheral iridectomy.

Figure 4–10. Pressure on the posterior lip of the wound prolapses iris tissue. This generally is accomplished quite easily, since the incision for a surgical sector iridectomy is somewhat larger than that for a surgical peripheral iridectomy.

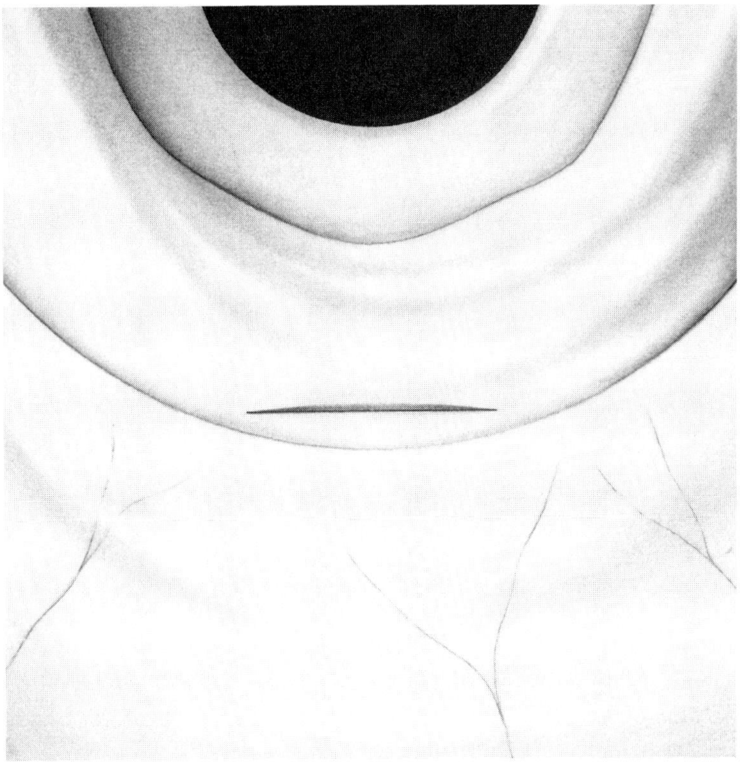

Figure 4–9

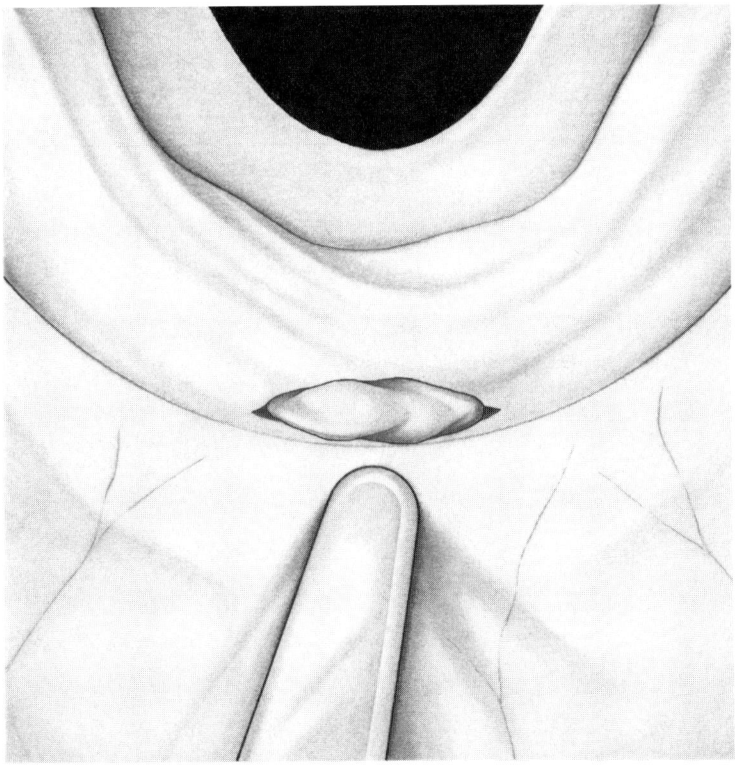

Figure 4–10

Figure 4–11. The tissue is grasped and gently withdrawn with a hand-over-hand technique until the sphincter is present at the wound edge.

Figure 4–12. Once the sphincter is seen at the edge of the wound, it is excised in a cordlike fashion to create an iridectomy.

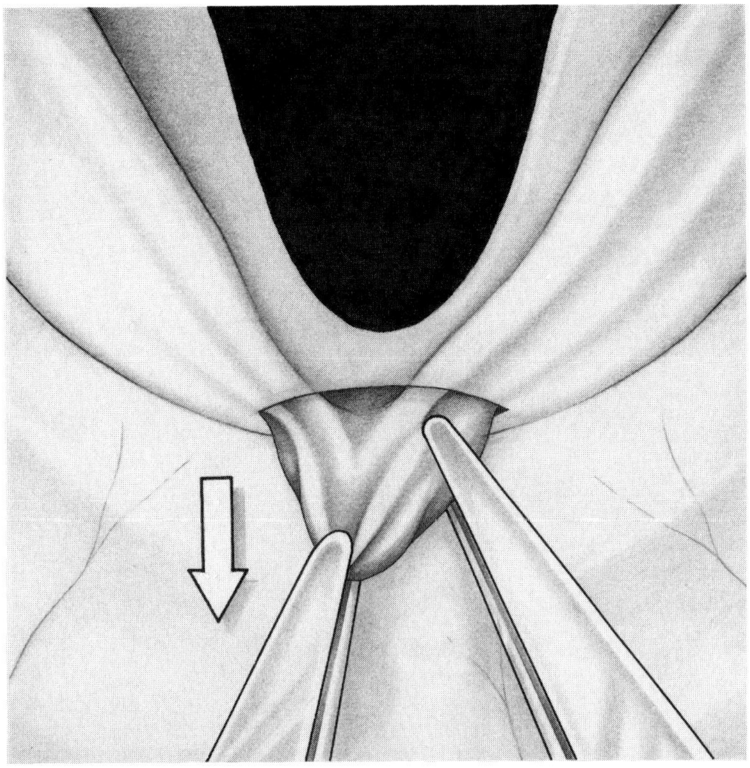
Figure 4–11

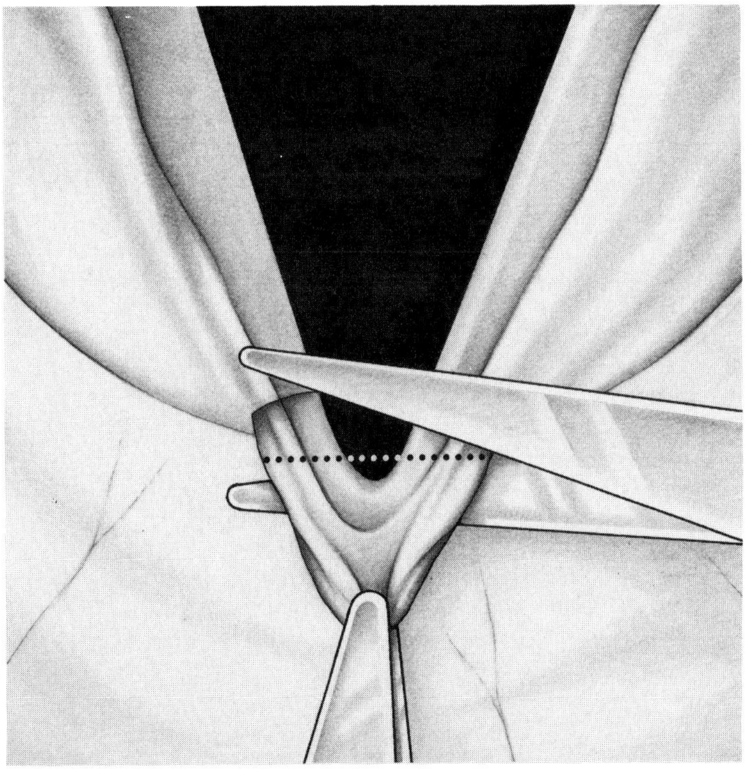
Figure 4–12

Figure 4–13. Alternately, a three-step incision can be made, which makes a slightly narrower iridectomy.

Figure 4–14. The incision is closed with a single 10-0 nylon suture.

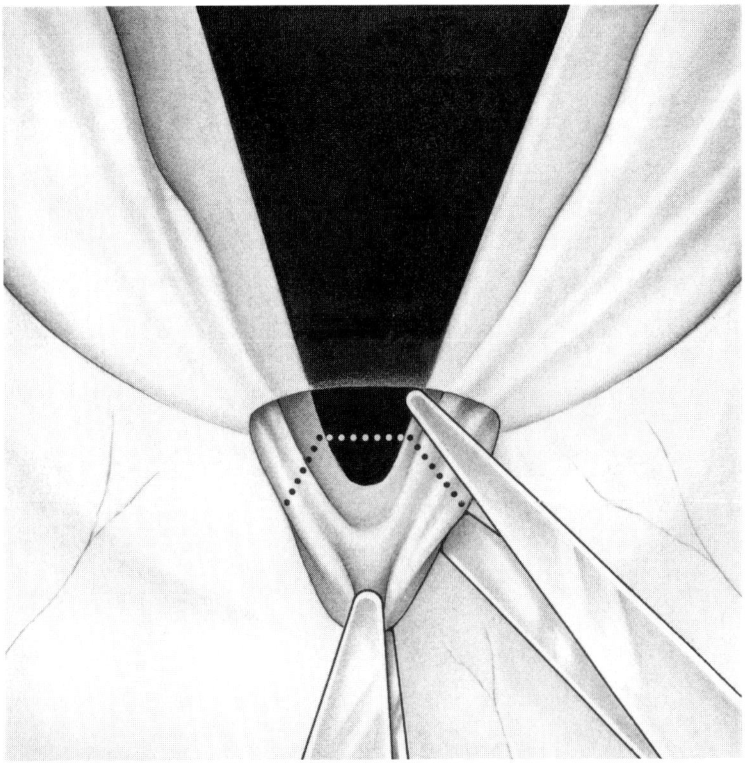

Figure 4–13

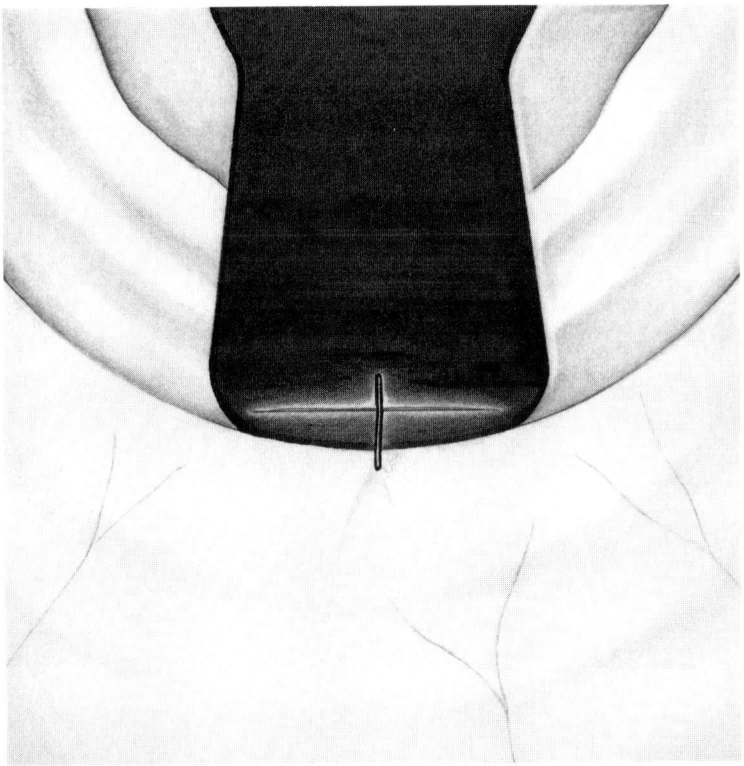

Figure 4–14

5

Laser Trabeculoplasty

The principle of argon laser trabeculoplasty is to alter the configuration of the trabecular meshwork to enhance aqueous outflow. There is a variety of indications for this procedure, but for the most part, it is reserved for those conditions where control of glaucoma is difficult by medically tolerated means, but surgical intervention is not yet appropriate. In effect, this procedure buys time in managing the chronic disease. It is also a helpful adjunct in aging patients who have maturing cataracts, in whom a miotic agent would produce exaggerated visual difficulties. Although there are several published studies examining the use of argon laser trabeculoplasty as a primary procedure, in most instances, it is used in concert with medical treatment.

Figure 5–1. Laser trabeculoplasty is best performed where there is a good view of the filtration angle. It is, therefore, desirable to have a reasonably clear cornea and an adequate gonioscopic view of the angle structures. In some instances, these may be a prominent last roll of the iris in an eye with open-angle glaucoma or appositional closure associated with combined-mechanism disease. In the first case, gonioplasty (see Chapter 3) is performed in the designated area prior to laser trabeculoplasty, whereas in the latter case, a laser peripheral iridectomy (see Chapter 3) may be desirable before the trabeculoplasty. In each circumstance, the angle is widened so that the structures are clearly visualized and treatable with laser energy.

An antireflective, coated, three-mirror Goldmann contact lens is used to separate the lids, stabilize the globe, act as a heat sink, and direct laser energy to the trabeculum. I generally choose to threat the inferior 180 degrees of the angle as the primary area. Should further treatment be required, the superior half of the angle circumference can be treated at a second session.

The three-mirror lens is inserted between the lids to a topically anesthetized cornea. Since I turn the lens clockwise as I treat the angle, I place the goniomirror in the horizontal position that permits access to the portion of the angle I choose to treat. As indicated, when the mirror is on the left, the inferior angle is treated. When one wants to treat the superior angle, the mirror is initially positioned to the right. By doing this, there is little confusion on how to rotate the lens as the treatment progresses.

Figure 5–2. The argon laser energy is delivered perpendicular to the mirror to strike the trabeculum. It is preferable to treat the anterior portion of the trabecular meshwork to achieve the maximal effect. The beam should be attenuated and focused precisely before the foot pedal is depressed. Specific focusing will permit the optimal amount of energy to be delivered.

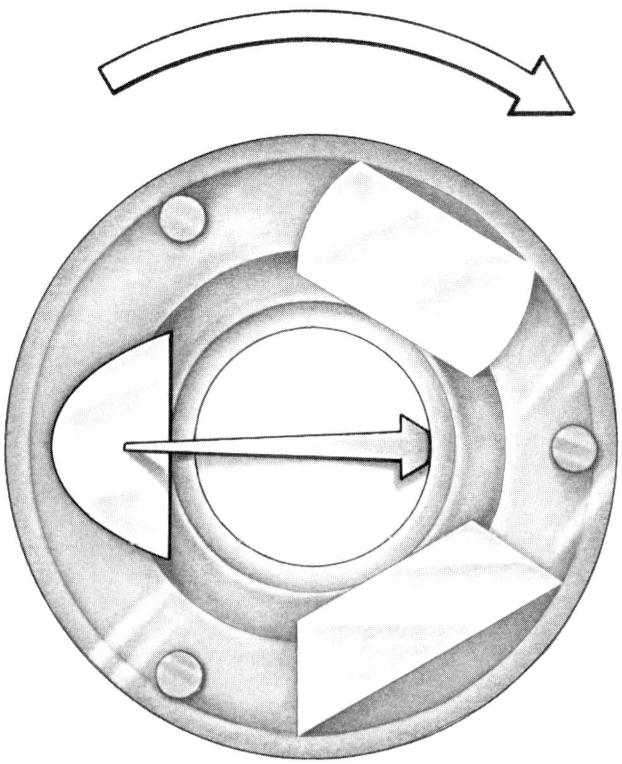

Figure 5–1

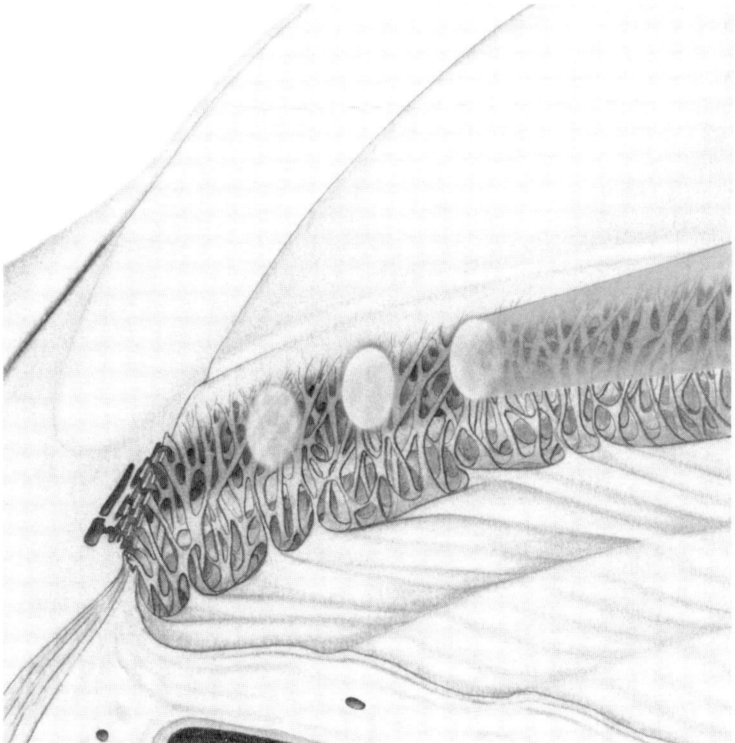

Figure 5–2

Figure 5–3. The settings for argon laser trabeculoplasty fall within a fairly tight range, with power settings varying between 750 and 1000 mW, depending on the quality of the laser burn on the trabecular tissue. A 50-μm spot size at a 0.2 second delivery commonly is used. The amount of energy is adjusted depending on the appearance of the tissue reaction.

1. Blanching of the pigment in the trabeculum indicates that an adequate take has occurred.
2. If there is no evidence of a take, there is inadequate energy delivery or tissue absorption; since we cannot influence tissue absorption, the energy setting is increased until a tissue reaction occurs.
3. At times, blanching will be accompanied by a gas bubble, which suggests that this is the upper limit of energy required.
4. A burned or charred area indicates that too great an amount of energy is provided, and the setting should be reduced.

One should note that the angle pigmentation varies around the circumference of the trabeculum and that there often is greater pigmentation in the inferior angle as opposed to the upper angle. There may even be variation between the angle and the horizontal meridia with relation to the angle at 6 o'clock. Therefore, it is possible that variations in the amount of energy must be adjusted during the procedure.

Figure 5–4. The major considerations in performing a laser trabeculoplasty successfully are the amount of energy delivered and the site of delivery. Since the goniolens is used to visualize the angle, the surgeon must be certain that he or she identifies the landmarks. As I have indicated, the most desirable area of treatment is the anterior trabeculum or the junction of Schlemm's canal and the trabecular meshwork. At times, the posterior trabeculum is treated when the anatomy is not precisely visible. This probably will be effective but runs the risk of putting burns in the ciliary body, a more posterior structure. Burns placed in the ciliary body will not be effective in reducing the IOP, will increase inflammation, and might lead to synechia formation. If possible, this posterior area of treatment should be avoided.

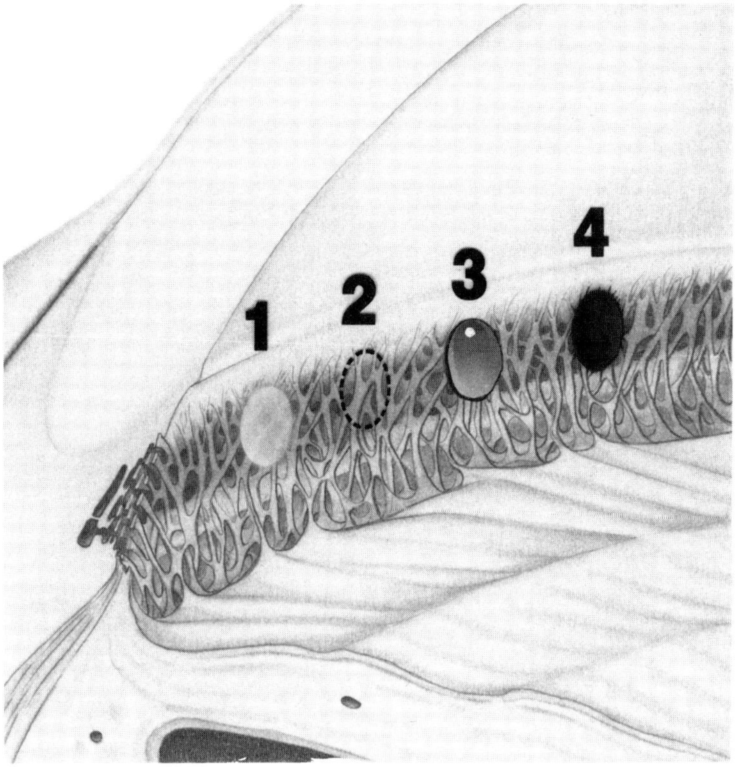

Figure 5–3

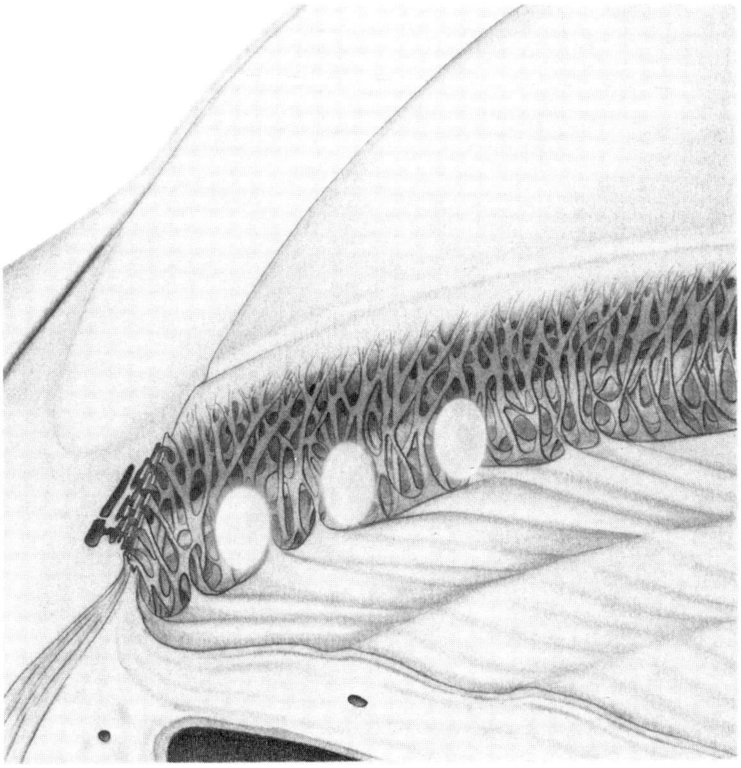

Figure 5–4

Figure 5–5. Laser burns to the iris substance also should be avoided. At times, the patient's eye or head may move while the laser is activated, and an iris burn may occur under these conditions. It is important to instruct the patient regarding the need to remain as immobile as possible during this procedure. In other situations, there may be a prominent last roll of the iris or areas of appositional closure. To prevent iris burns and to gain access to the angle, either gonioplasty or laser peripheral iridectomy can be performed, as we previously discussed.

Figure 5–6. Laser burns that are placed too anteriorly will result in delivery of energy to the corneal endothelium. Since this is a discrete burn, little damage will occur if the surgeon recognizes the situation promptly and makes the proper adjustment. Needless to say, a corneal burn will not reduce IOP.

In the proper setting, laser trabeculoplasty is a highly effective adjunct in reducing IOP. Fortunately, there is little morbidity in a properly performed procedure. There is a risk of elevating the IOP, producing inflammation, and causing tissue damage in cases that are imprecisely or too exuberantly done, so caution should be observed.

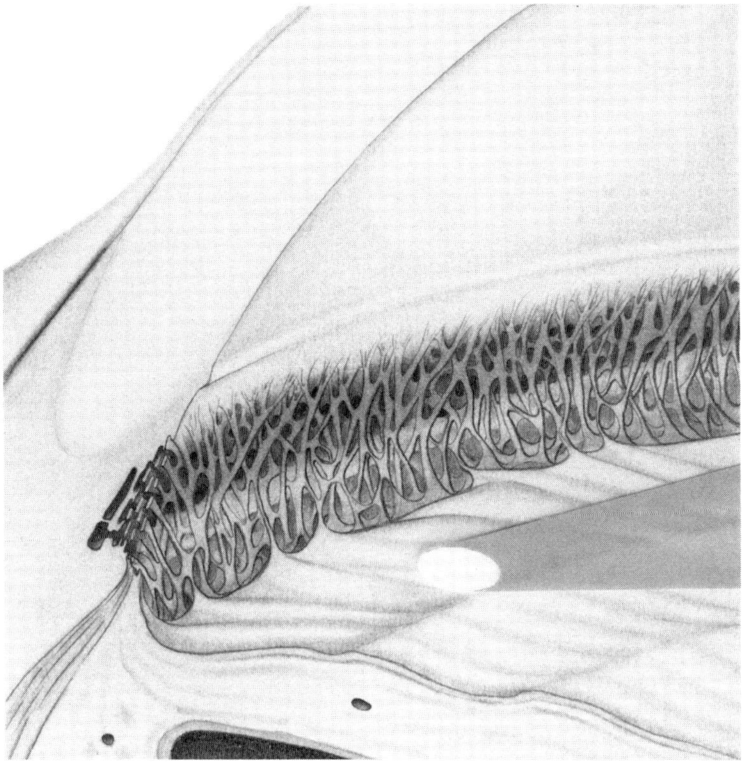

Figure 5–5

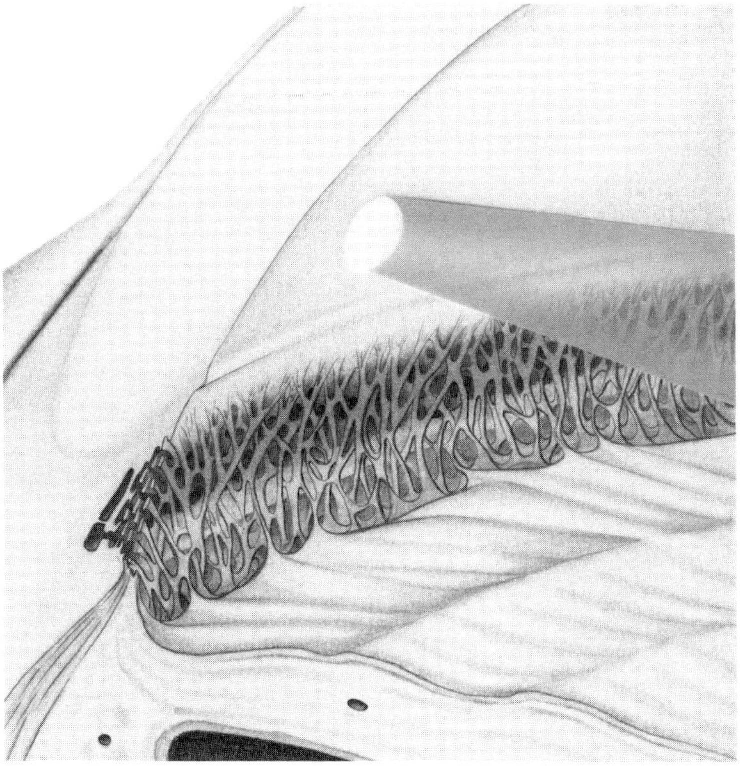

Figure 5–6

6

Trabecular Surgery

Trabeculectomy is a term that has been applied to a variety of procedures whose common feature is a sclerostomy performed under a lamellar scleral flap. In the illustrations in this chapter, I describe the procedure I prefer, along with several alternative operations.

Figure 6–1. A paracentesis is made through clear cornea. This site will be used to inject Healon or saline should it be necessary to reform the anterior chamber at the completion of the procedure.

Figure 6–2. A conjunctival flap is mobilized to expose the corneoscleral limbus. I prefer the limbal-based conjunctival flap, since I believe it offers the optimal protection to the filtration site. Incision in the conjunctival tissue starts to one side of the superior rectus tendon. The Tenon's layer is then grasped and incised to the sclera. A foamy layer is then apparent. Blunt dissection is performed in this anatomic plane to expose the conjunctival–corneal junction.

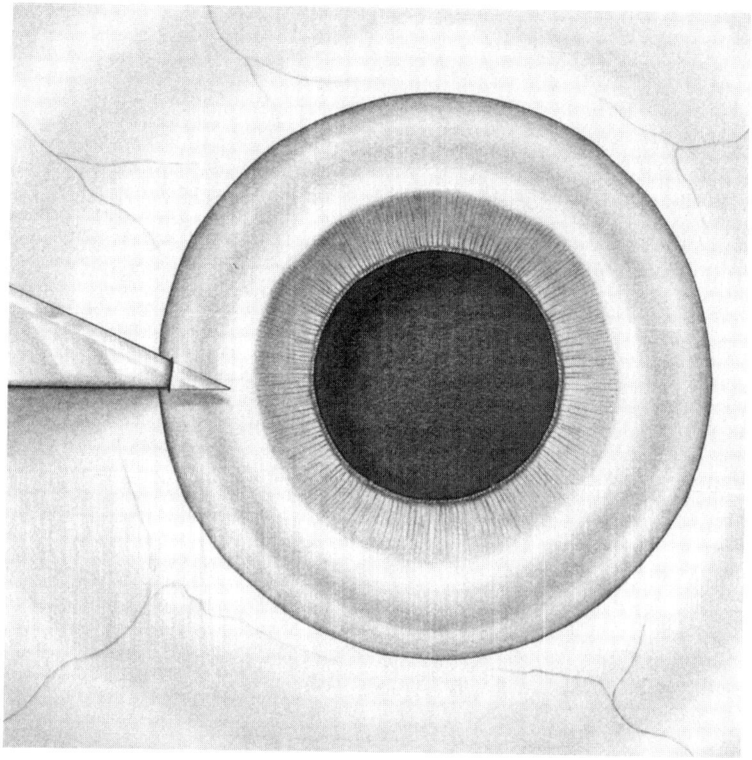

Figure 6–1

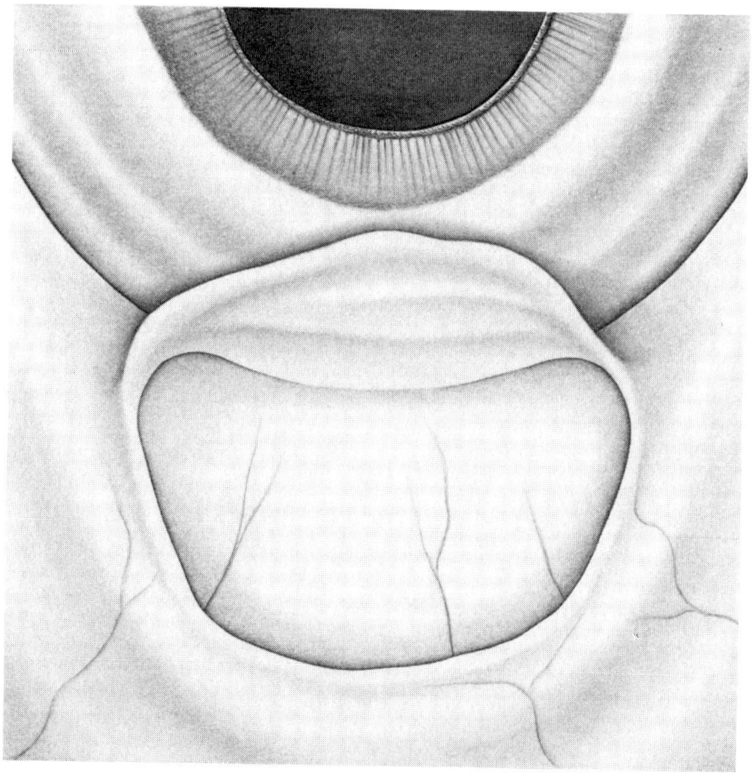

Figure 6–2

Figure 6–3. Alternately, a fornix-based flap can be prepared. The conjunctival–Tenon's layer is incised at the corneoscleral limbus with dissection superiorly toward the superior rectus muscle. An advantage of a fornix-based flap is that it reduces the chance of buttonholing the conjunctiva.

Figure 6–4. Another method to expose the corneoscleral limbus modifies the fornix-based scleral flap. This triangular flap facilitates apposition of the tissues at the completion of the procedure.

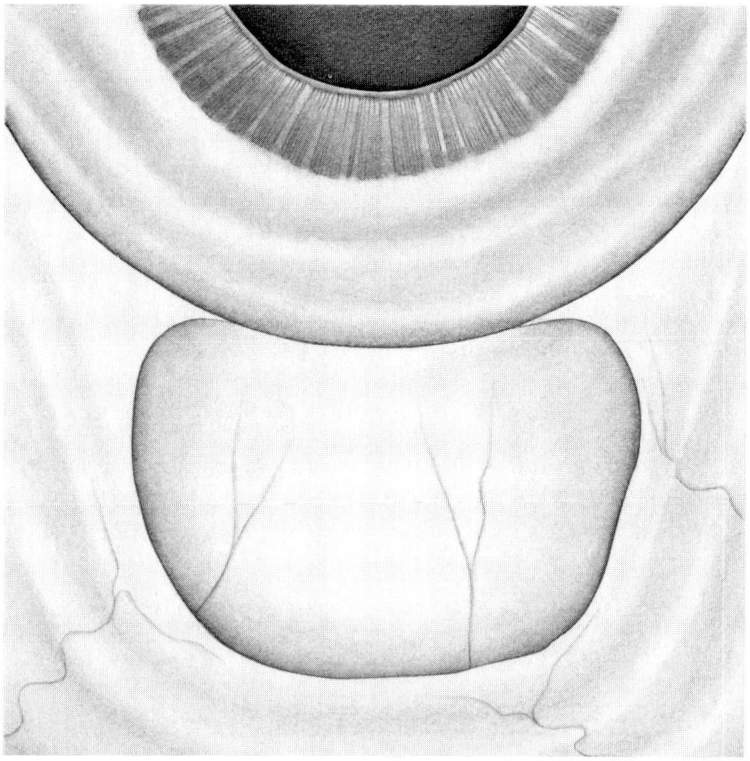

Figure 6–3

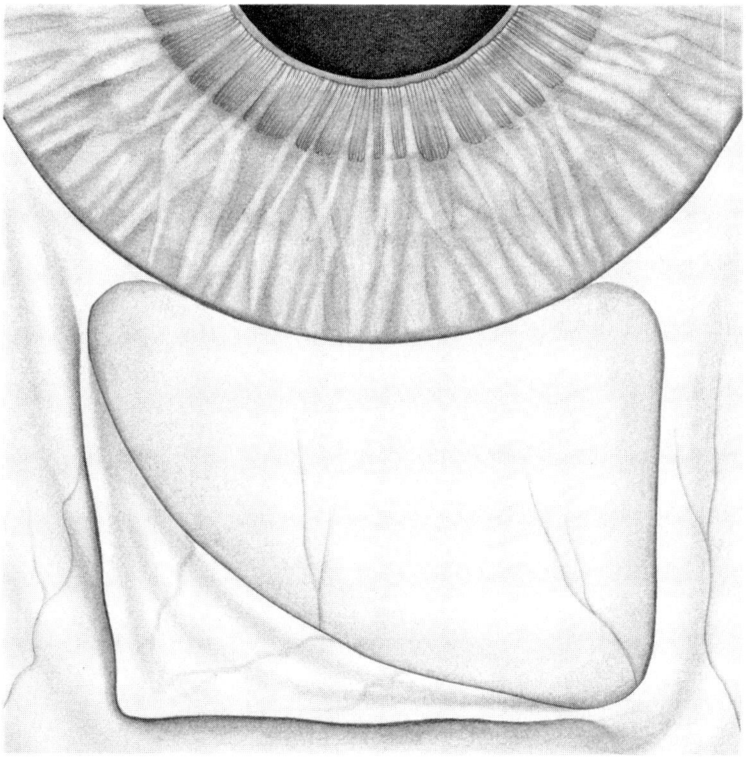

Figure 6–4

Figure 6–5. The superficial scleral tissue is treated with the bipolar hemostatic eraser. This cauterizes superficial vessels and creates a clean scleral surface. It also permits identification of remnants of Tenon's capsule that have not been reflected.

Figure 6–6. A rectangular superficial scleral flap is then prepared by sharp dissection. The dimensions of the rectangle are approximately 4×4 mm, and its base is at the limbus. The depth of dissection is approximately one third to one half of scleral thickness. The dissection can be performed with a diamond blade or with a Paufique-type metal blade. Gentle upward traction is placed on the flap to stretch the scleral fibers for a smooth dissection. As the limbus is approached, the orientation of the dissection is altered to follow the contour of the globe. Otherwise, the flap becomes extremely thinned anteriorly and may tear. It has been my impression that a flap of this type promotes better drainage than does a thicker one.

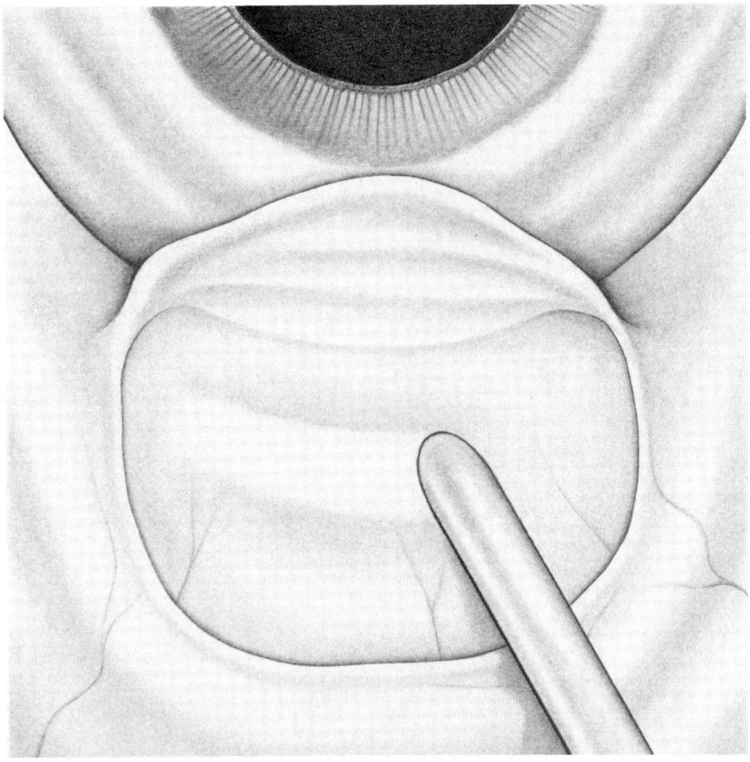

Figure 6–5

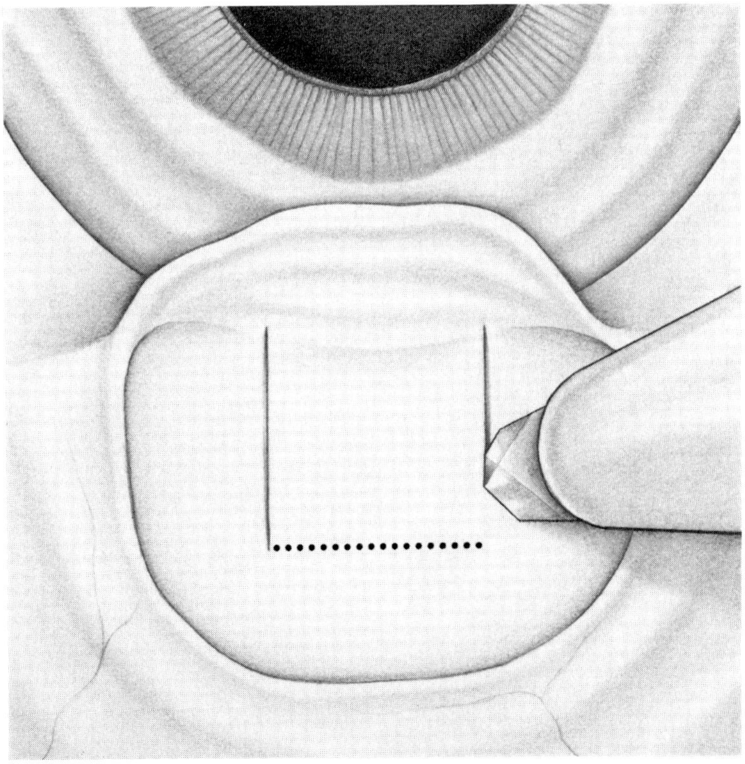

Figure 6–6

Figure 6–7. A triangular flap can be fashioned as an alternative. This type of scleral dissection is closed with a single suture at its apex.

Figure 6–8. Dissection of the superficial scleral flap is continued anteriorly into clear corneal tissue. In preparing the superficial scleral dissection, the perpendicular limbs of the incisions should be carried forward to the reflection of the conjunctival–corneal junction, which is demarcated by a bump in the tissue. The tip of the blade should be visible in clear cornea when the conjunctival flap is reflected to its initial position. The anterior extent of the dissection facilitates subsequent removal of the deeper block of scleral tissue later in the procedure.

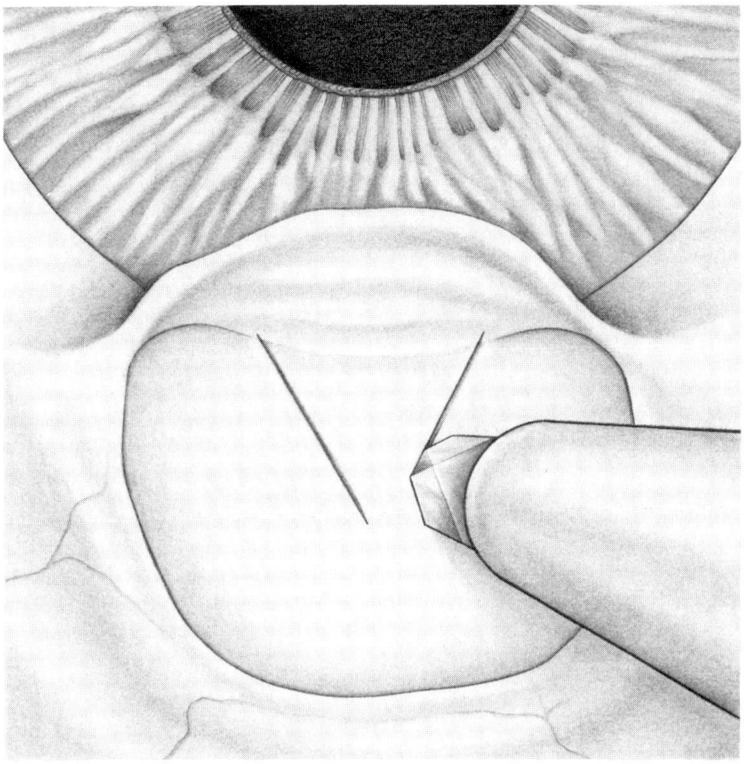

Figure 6–7

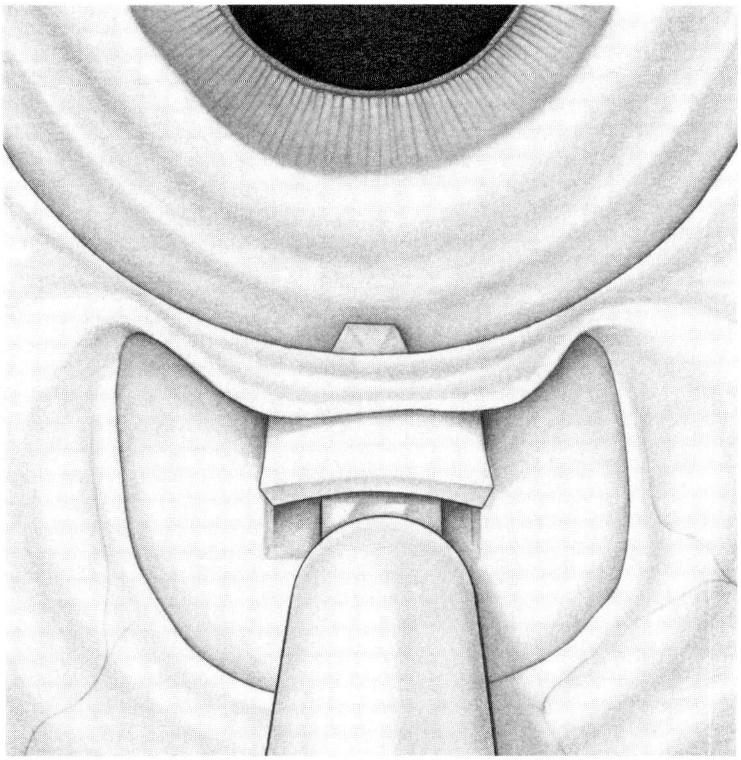

Figure 6–8

Figure 6–9. A cross-sectional view shows that the superficial lamellar dissection starts posteriorly in the sclera about 4 mm from the conjunctival–corneal junction and is continued anteriorly into clear cornea. The anterior aspect of this lamellar preparation actually is forward of the trabecular meshwork.

Figure 6–10. When the trabeculectomy procedure is performed behind the scleral spur, the safest and easiest way to enter the superchoroidal space is to use a cautery or diathermy to penetrate the deep scleral tissues 3–3.5 mm behind the limbus. The cautery is applied in a sequential fashion at a single site in deep sclera. As soon as a color change to deep gray or brown is seen, the cauterization should be stopped.

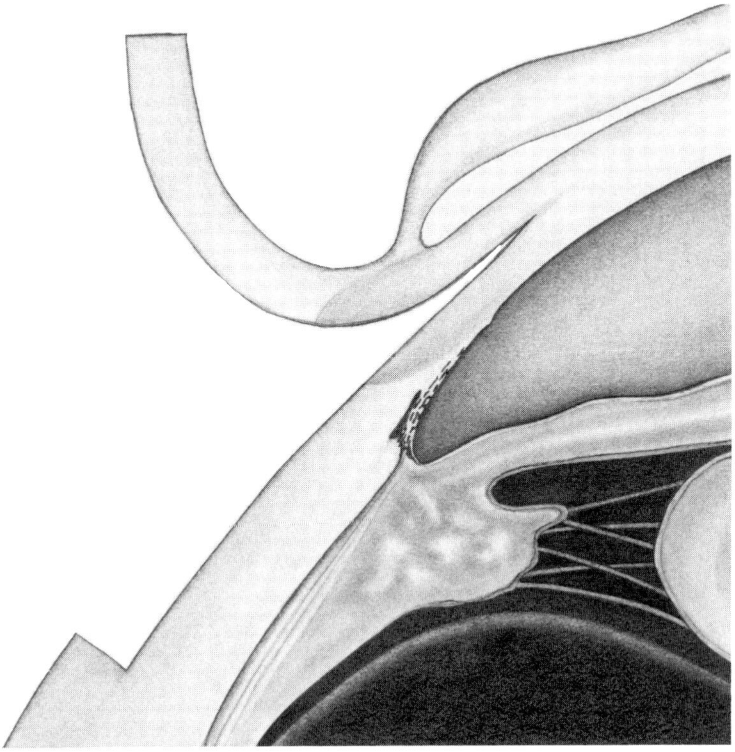

Figure 6–9

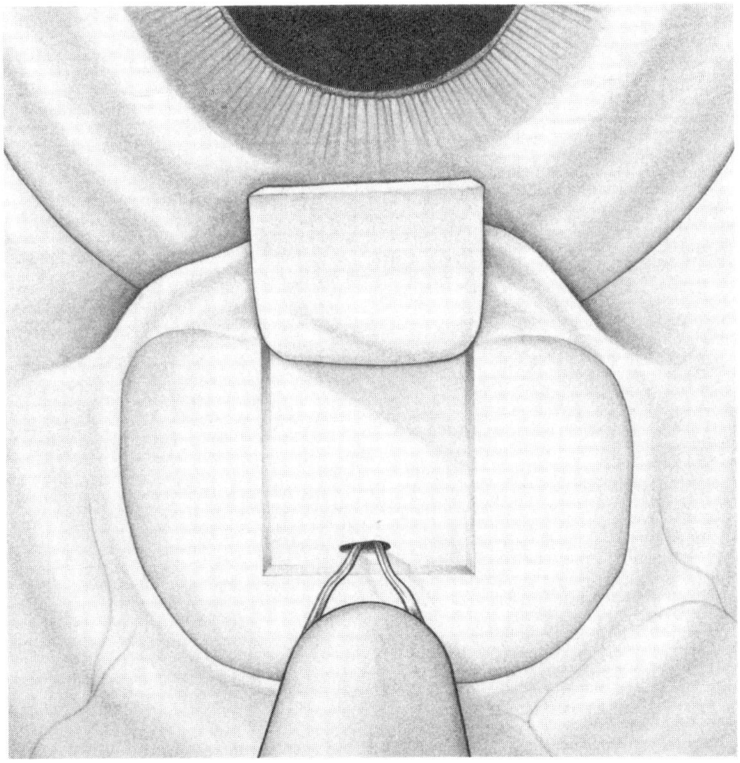

Figure 6–10

Figure 6–11. The cross-sectional representation indicates the cautery entry through the deeper scleral tissue into the superchoroidal space overlying the ciliary body.

Figure 6–12. One blade of a blunt-tipped scissors is then inserted into the cautery entry to enlarge the incision parallel to the limbus, almost to the full extent of the lamellar bed on each side. The incision is extended to the margins of the lamellar dissection, since as large a block of tissue that can be excised should be removed. The two incisions perpendicular to the limbus are made with the tips of the scissors pointed upward to avoid damaging the ciliary body. The forward extent of the excisions is the junction of the conjunctival–corneal tissues. The superficial scleral flap protects against buttonholing the conjunctiva.

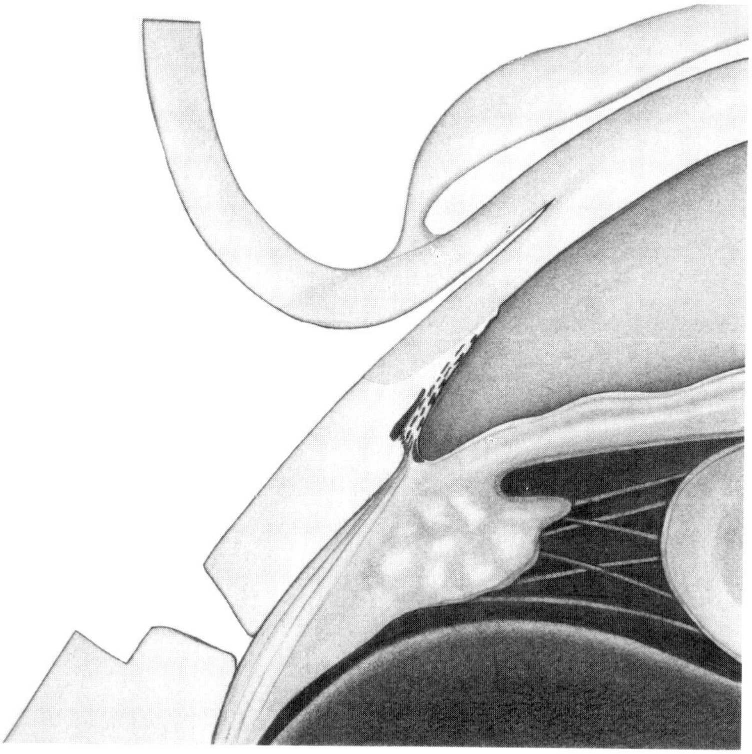

Figure 6–11

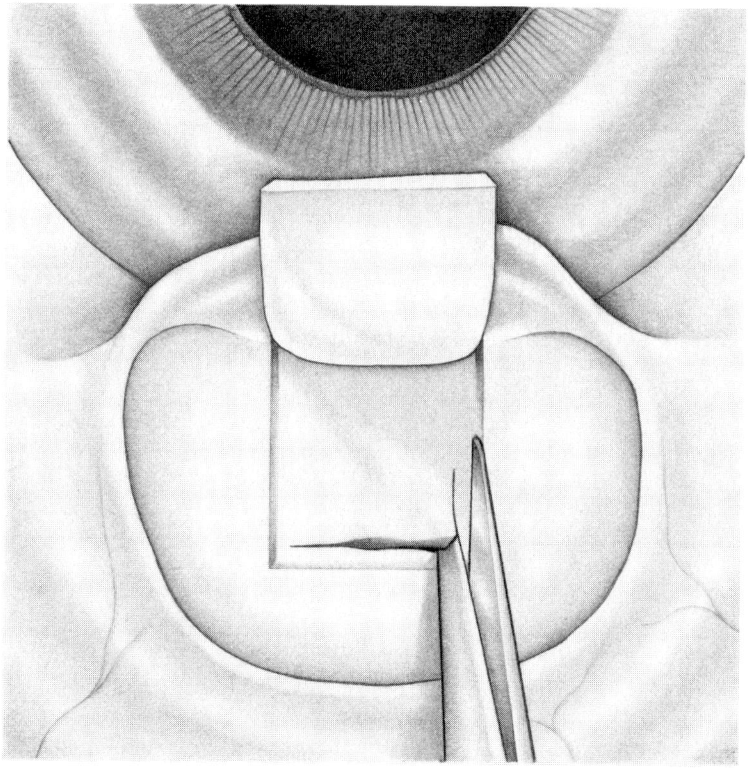

Figure 6–12

Figure 6–13. The deep scleral tissue is separated from the underlying ciliary body using a rounded, dull spatula. This separation is accomplished by elevating the scleral flap with one hand while gently teasing the fine bridging fibers from the posterior aspect of the sclera.

Figure 6–14. The tissue separation in the superchoroidal space is continued anteriorly until the scleral spur is disinserted and the anterior chamber is entered. In patients using chronic miotic drugs, there may be a significant membranous reaction, with consequent thickening of the scleral spur. Extreme caution should be exercised during the disinsertion to avoid stripping Descemet's membrane or causing hemorrhage from fine vessels.

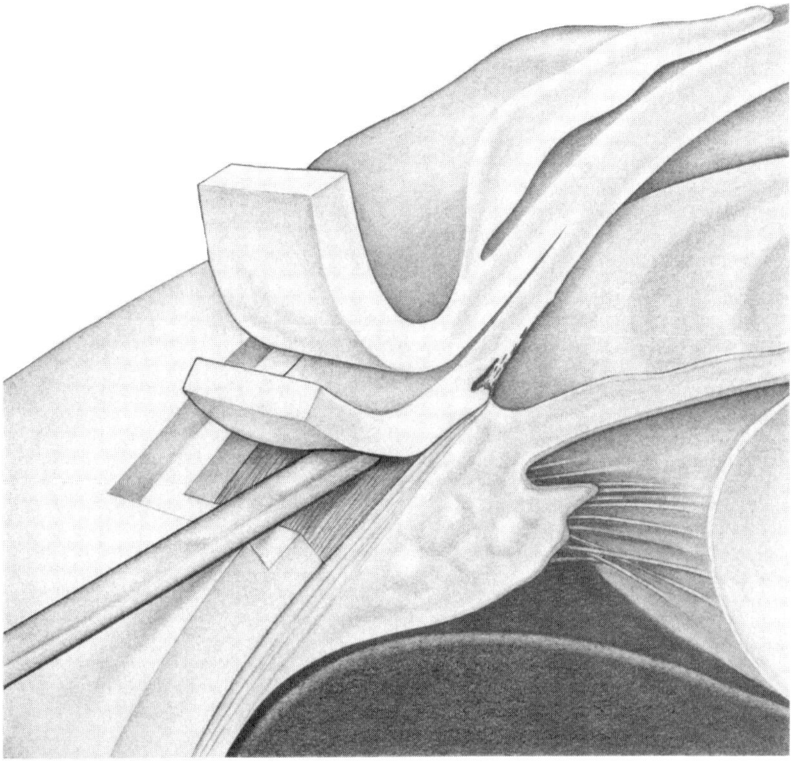

Figure 6–13

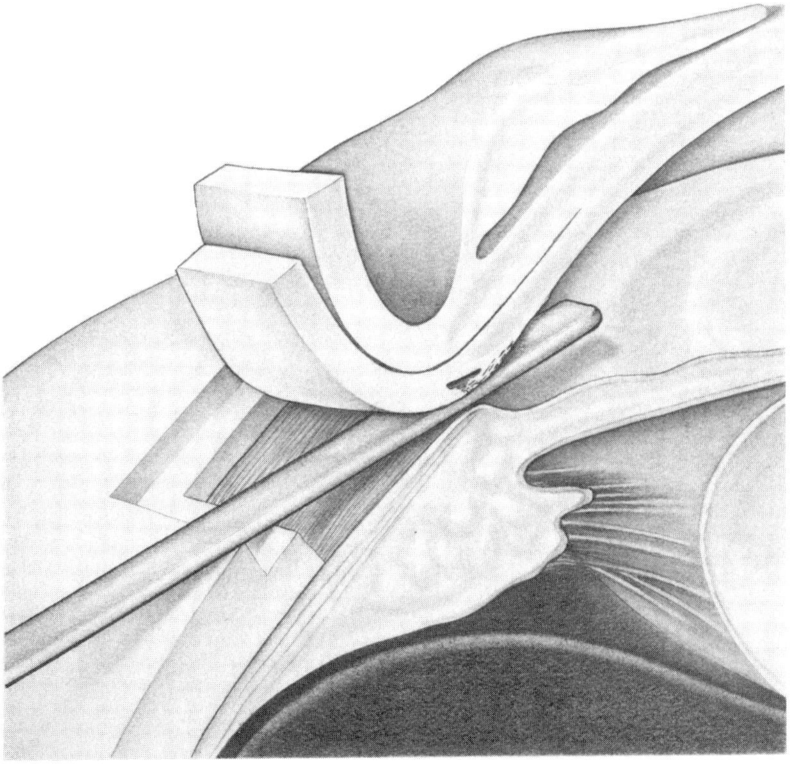

Figure 6–14

Figure 6–15. The deep scleral flap, having been mobilized from the underlying ciliary body, is attached only in its corneal aspect. Excision of this block of tissue containing cornea, trabecular meshwork, and sclera is done with scissors as far anteriorly in the cornea as possible. The reason the superficial scleral flap is carried into clear cornea (see Figs. 6–8 and 6–9) is to facilitate this excision.

Figure 6–16. The iridectomy should be as wide as the internal ostium of the trabeculectomy. If it is too small, as aqueous passes through it, the iris will be forced against the trabeculectomy site and eventually will seal the opening. Care must be exercised to avoid damaging the crystalline lens. In addition, too much traction on the iris can result in an iridodialysis and bleeding.

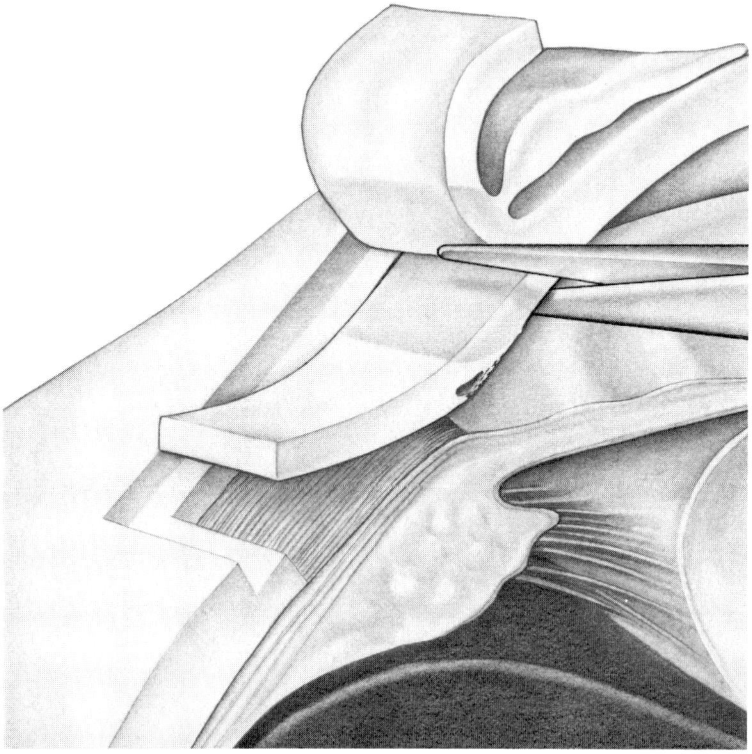

Figure 6–15

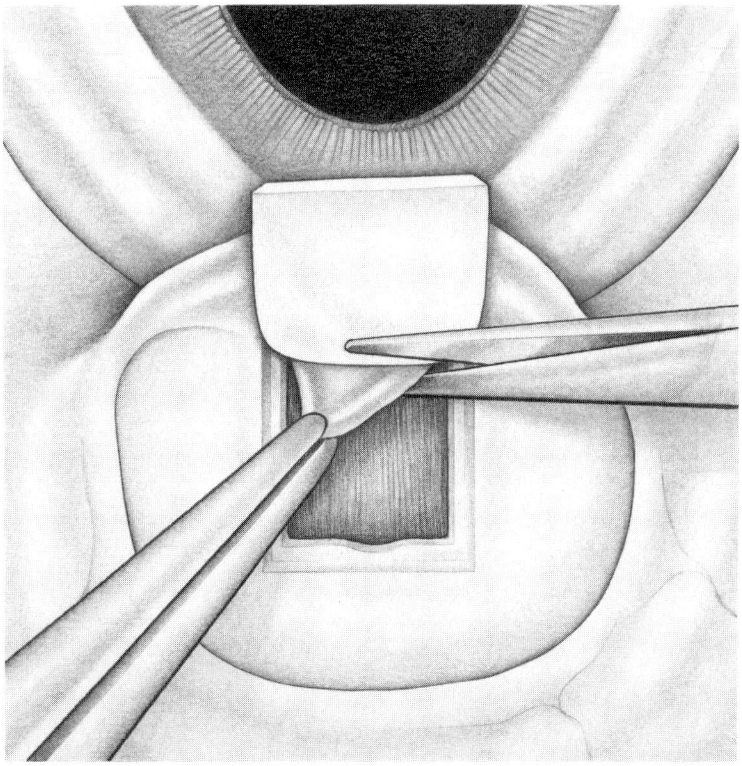

Figure 6–16

Figure 6–17. The lamellar scleral flap is closed at its superior corners with 10-0 nylon sutures. The flap is reapposed to its proper anatomic site without tying the sutures too tightly.

Figure 6–18. The cross-sectional view of the procedure shows the deep block of excised tissue, including cornea, trabeculum, and sclera. In effect, the dissection over the ciliary body produces a cyclodialysis, which adds to the pressure-reducing aspect of this particular procedure.

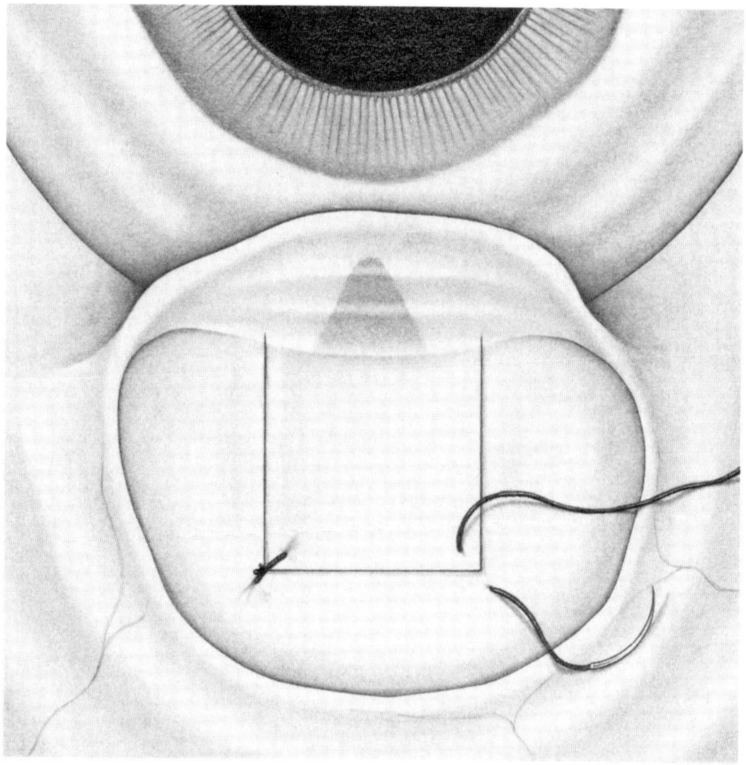

Figure 6–17

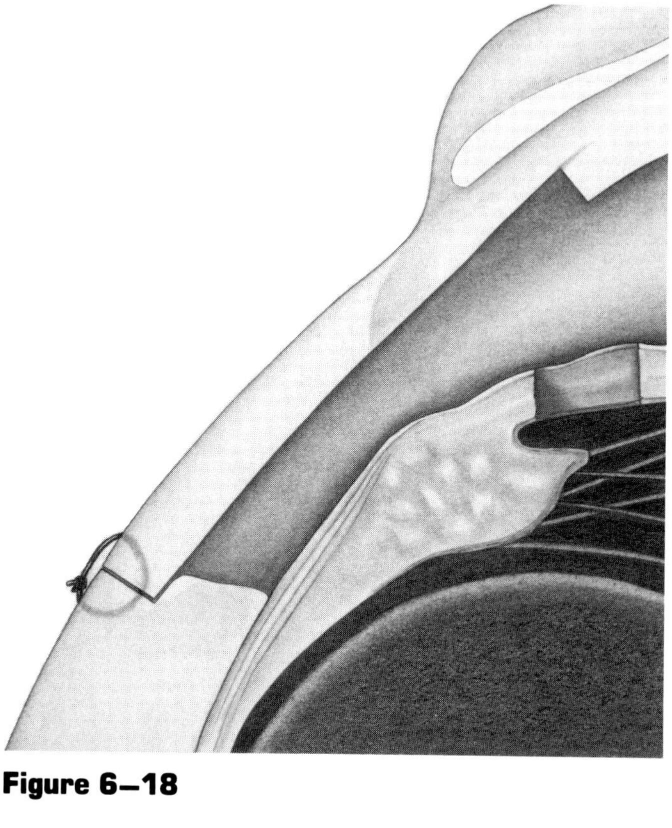

Figure 6–18

Figure 6–19. The conjunctival–Tenon's flap is closed in a continuous running fashion with an 8-0 or 9-0 Vicryl suture, being certain that both layers are included. If the Tenon's layer is particularly thickened and prominent, it can be carefully excised. Generally, with this technique, the anterior chamber is formed to some degree after completion of the procedure. When the chamber is very shallow or if it appears absent, either balanced saline solution or, preferably, a small amount of Healon is injected through the previously prepared paracentesis incision (see Fig. 6–1). The amount of Healon injected should simply fill out the chamber by flattening the iris. An excessive amount can produce slowing of aqueous flow through the filtering bleb.

Figure 6–20. A fornix-based conjunctival flap is closed by securing the edges of the flap to the clear cornea. The flap should be drawn down and be free of tension, or it will retract prematurely.

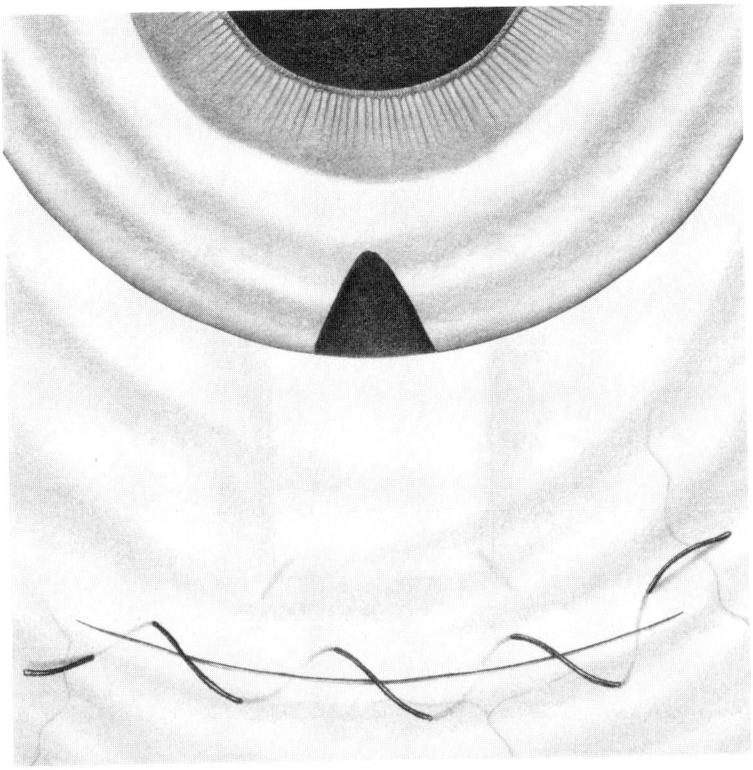

Figure 6–19

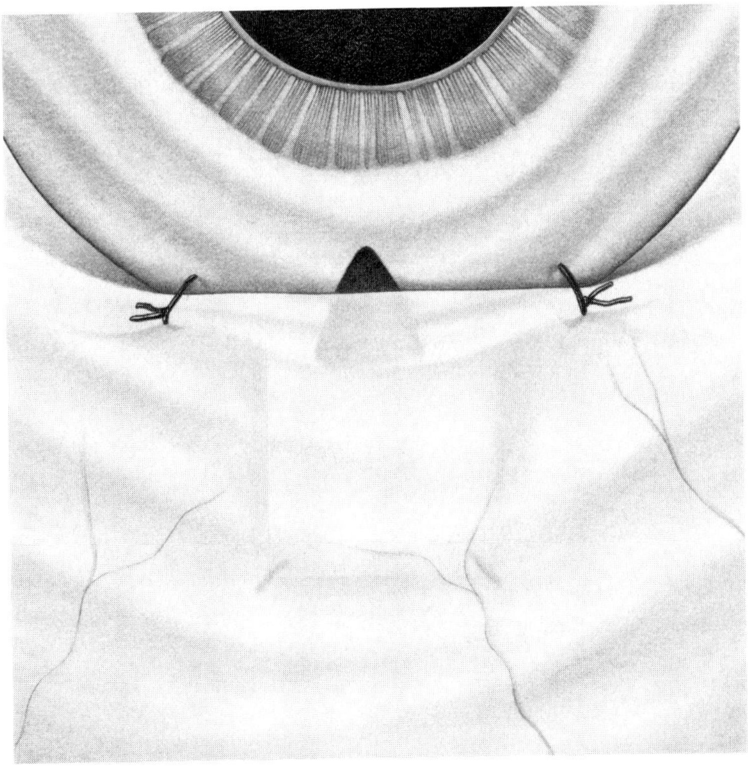

Figure 6–20

Figure 6–21. One advantage of a triangular-type conjunctival flap is that, in effect, a relaxing incision—the one perpendicular to the limbus—is made. When the incision is closed, there is little traction on the flap, and the chances of early retraction are remote. Once again, a single bite should include clear corneal tissue to secure the anterior portion of the flap.

Figure 6–22. When using the limbus-based flap, a buttonhole of the conjunctiva should be attended to during the procedure. The position and size of the buttonhole in this situation are less severe than one directly overlying the scleral dissection site in procedures performed under a scleral flap. This small dehiscence can be sutured directly with a figure-of-8 or mattress suture. Its edges should be compressed and inverted. The buttonhole is sutured on its inner aspect before conjunctival flap closure.

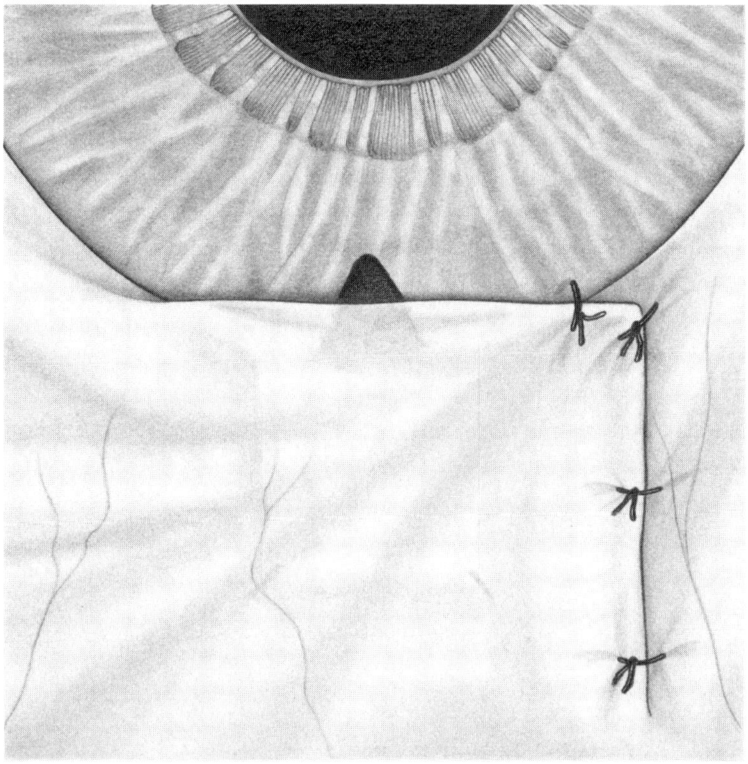

Figure 6–21

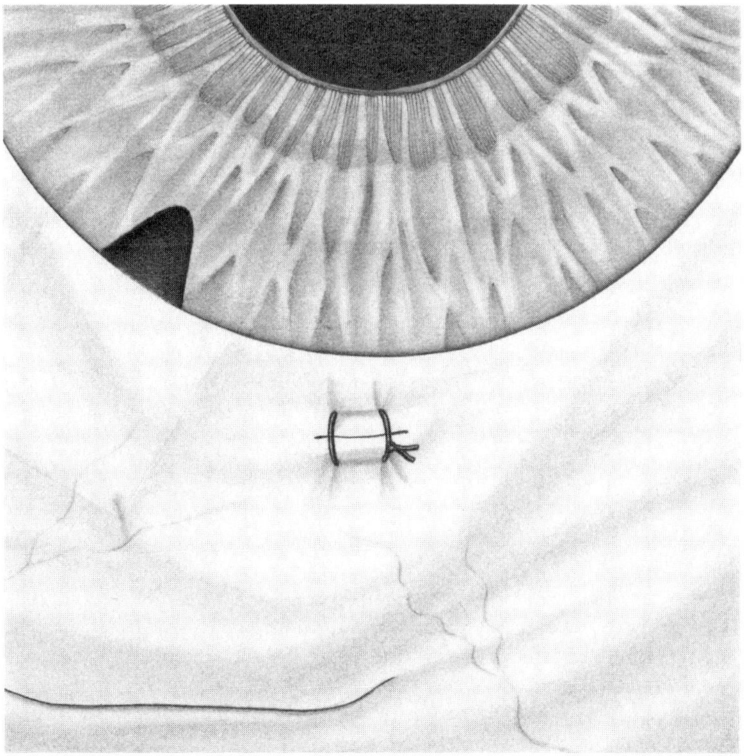

Figure 6–22

Figure 6–23. A discontinuity in the anterior edge of the superficial lamella occurs because the dissection is thinned in this area, and traction exerted during the procedure may tear it. Since it lies directly over the excised layer of sclera and serves a protective function, it should be repaired by direct suturing with a 10-0 nylon suture. The edges should be apposed without excessive traction.

Figure 6–24. An alternative for excising a block of tissue beneath the superficial scleral flap is to remove the tissue backward toward the scleral spur. Entry into the anterior chamber is made through clear cornea in the depth of the anteriormost aspect of the lamellar dissection. This incision is extended for almost the entire width of the superficial scleral flap.

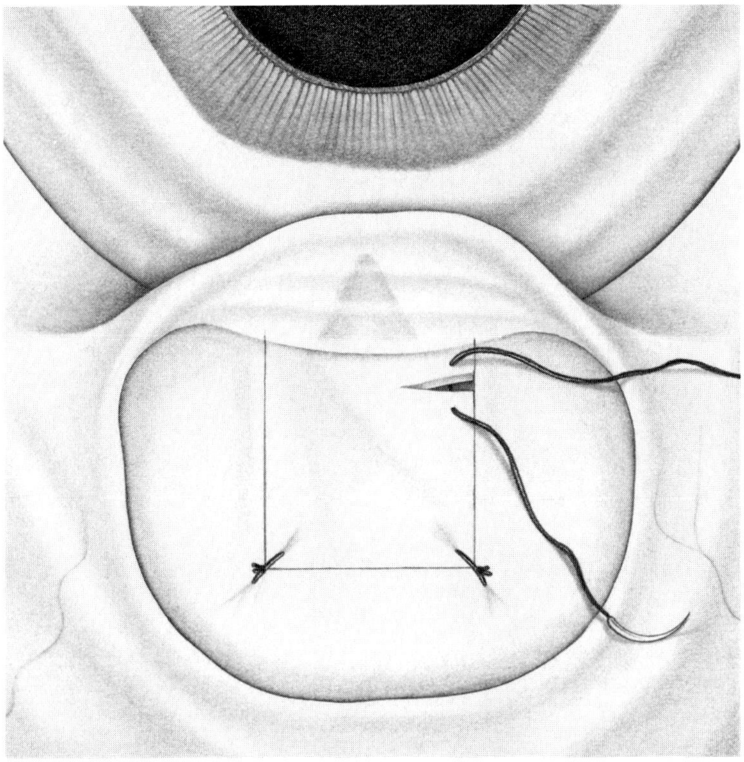

Figure 6–23

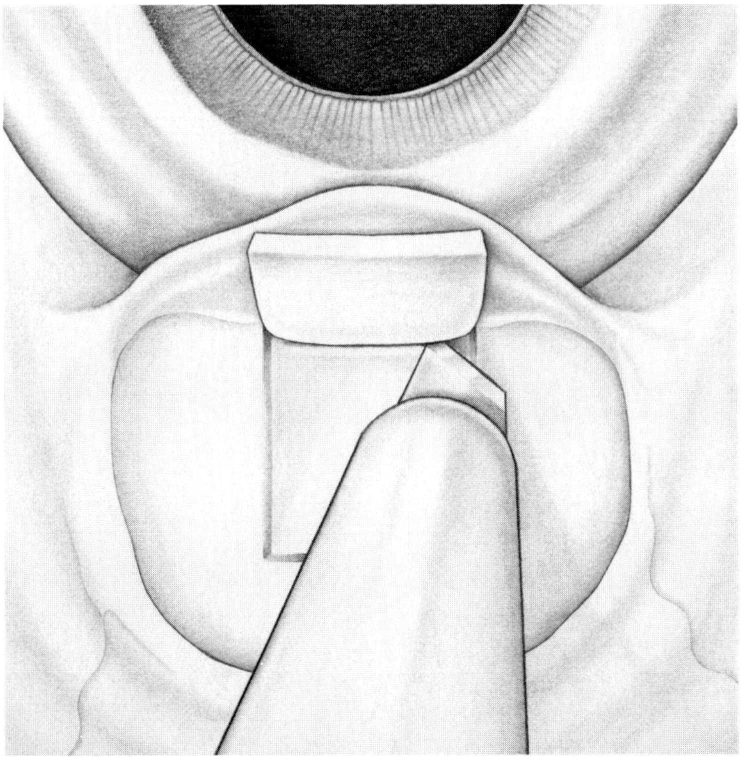

Figure 6–24

Figure 6–25. Using fine scissors, such as Vannas scissors, two radial incisions are made from the entry into the anterior chamber backward toward the scleral spur. The posterior lip of the corneoscleral wound is everted slightly to provide adequate visualization.

Figure 6–26. The entire block of tissue is excised parallel to the limbus. This section of tissue should contain peripheral cornea, trabeculum, and overlying sclera. The dissection remains anterior to the scleral spur. Once again, eversion of this posterior lip of tissue facilitates visualizing the extent of the excision. As in the technique described in Figure 6–16, an iridectomy at least the width of the sclerostomy site is performed.

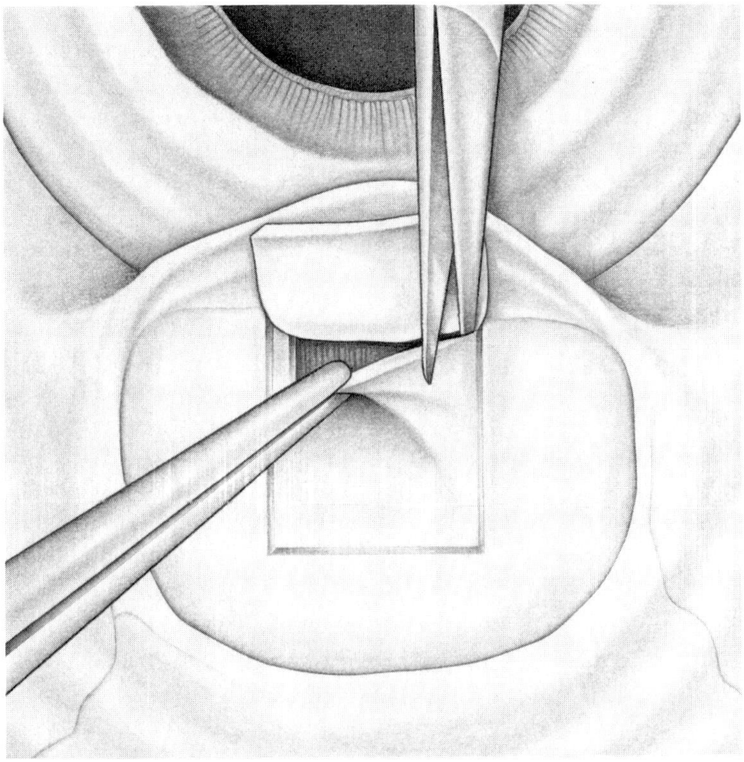

Figure 6–25

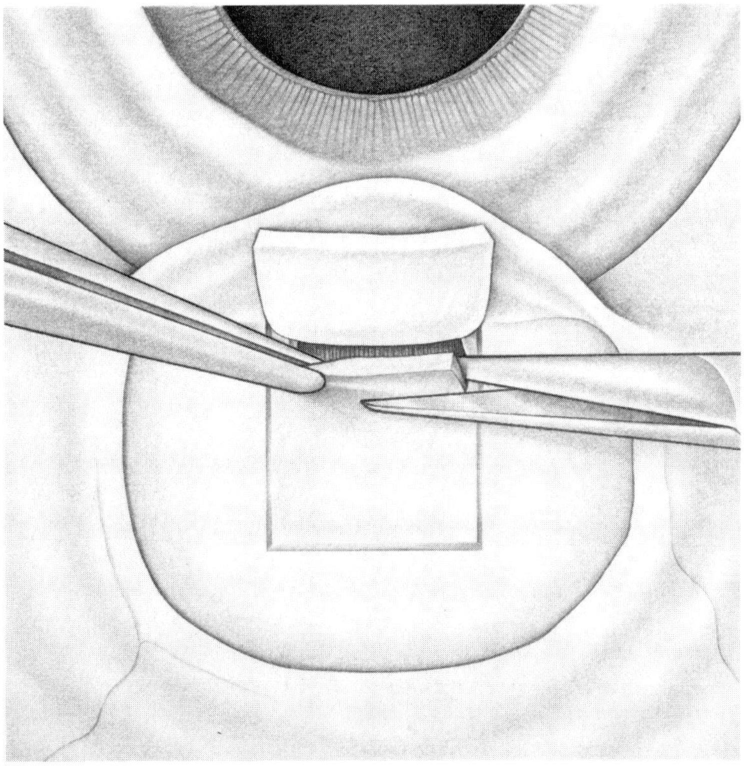

Figure 6–26

Figure 6–27. This cross-sectional view represents the condition when an anterior incision is made and not carried posteriorly. Although a piece of tissue beneath the scleral flap is excised, the trabeculum is not removed. Filtration may not necessarily occur in this situation.

Figure 6–28. The procedure described in Figure 6–24 will result in this appearance with excision of corneal, trabecular, and scleral tissue. The iridectomy is present to prevent occlusion of the sclerostomy site. The entire dissection is anterior to the scleral spur.

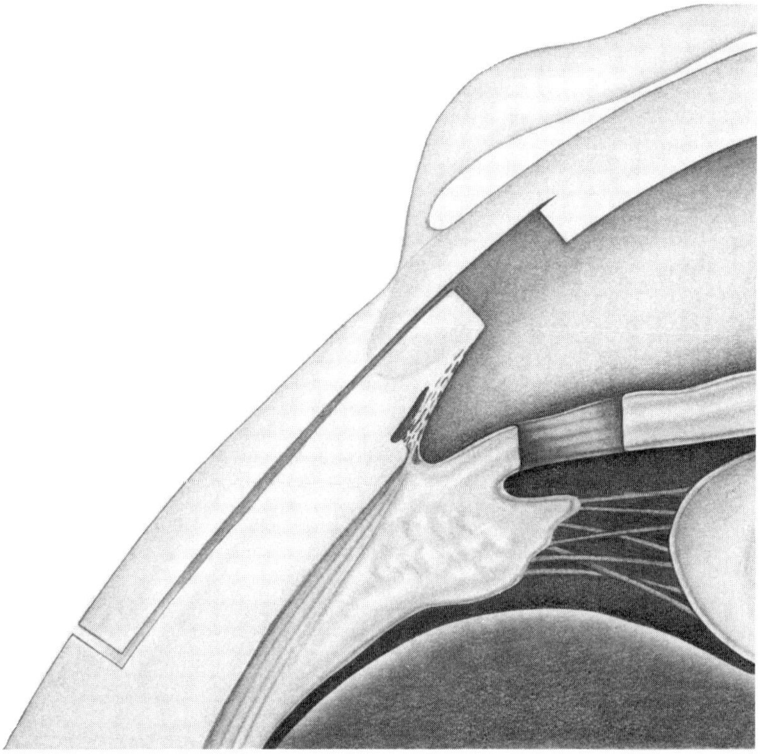

Figure 6–27

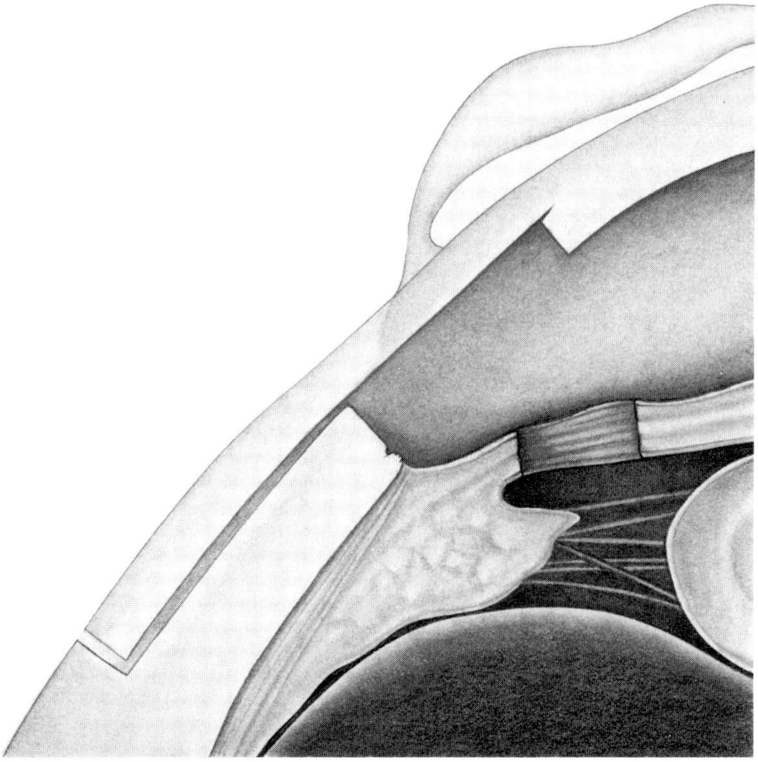

Figure 6–28

Figure 6–29. In the early postoperative period if the IOP begins to rise in the presence of a formed anterior chamber, gentle pressure placed adjacent to the bleb often will reduce the IOP and produce slight chamber shallowing. This sequence suggests that releasing the suture tension on the superficial sceral flap will induce greater filtration. The Hoskins lens is used to compress the conjunctival–Tenon's tissue overlying and surrounding the suture. The suture shards out prominently and can be lasered with either the argon or krypton laser. We use a 50–μm spot size, 200–300 mW of energy, and a pulse of short duration. We prefer using the krypton laser.

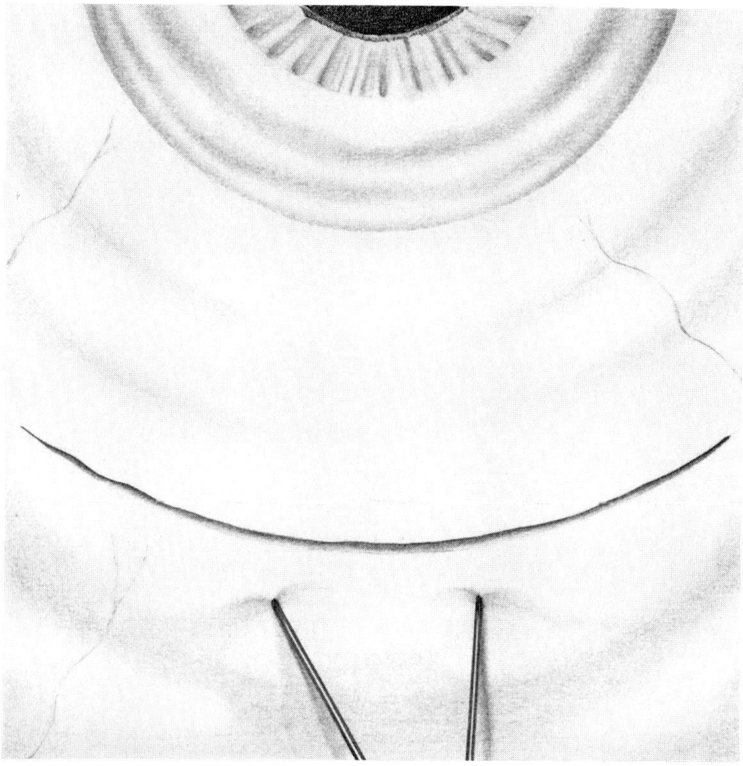

Figure 7–1

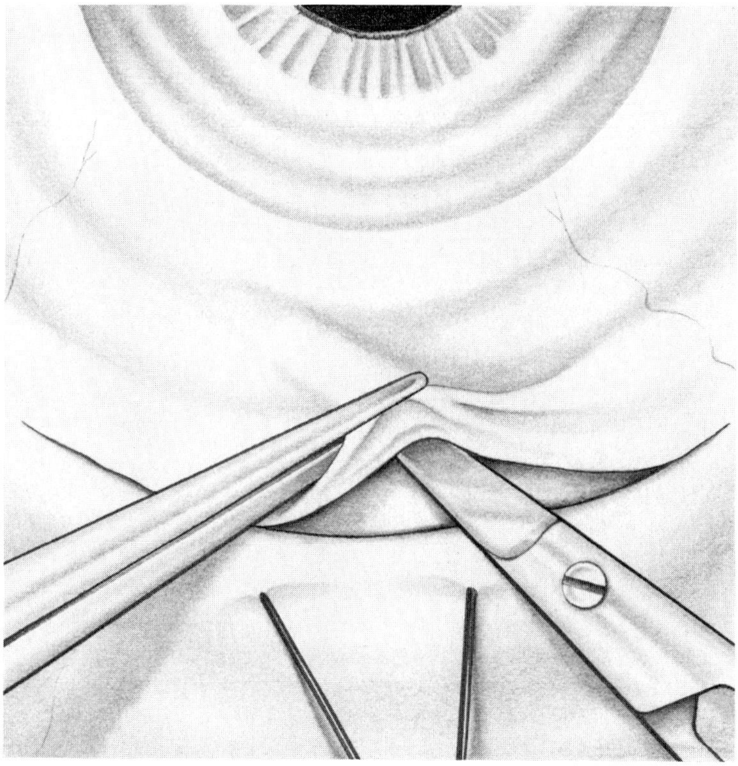

Figure 7–2

Figure 7–3. I have modified the classic Scheie procedure after the teaching of Dr. Bernard Becker, who suggested making a semilunar scleral flap and a superficial scleral lamellar dissection. This provides two advantages: first, the thermal burn penetrates through a thinner layer of tissue, and second, it protects the conjunctival–Tenon's tissue from the heating effects of the cautery. The base of the flap is at the reflection of the corneal and conjunctival epithelia.

Figure 7–4. The superficial lamellar dissection is approximately one third of scleral thickness and is carried anteriorly just to clear cornea. Identification of this landmark ensures that the entry will be into the anterior chamber. A disposable cautery is applied to the deeper layers of the sclera to create a line of contiguous burns running parallel to the limbus. The cautery is applied to make controlled burns, so that penetration of the tissue and entry into the anterior chamber does not occur prematurely. Aqueous contact with the cautery tip will cool it and obviate its further use. Should this occur, a scissors is inserted to complete the sclerostomy by incising the innermost layers of tissue.

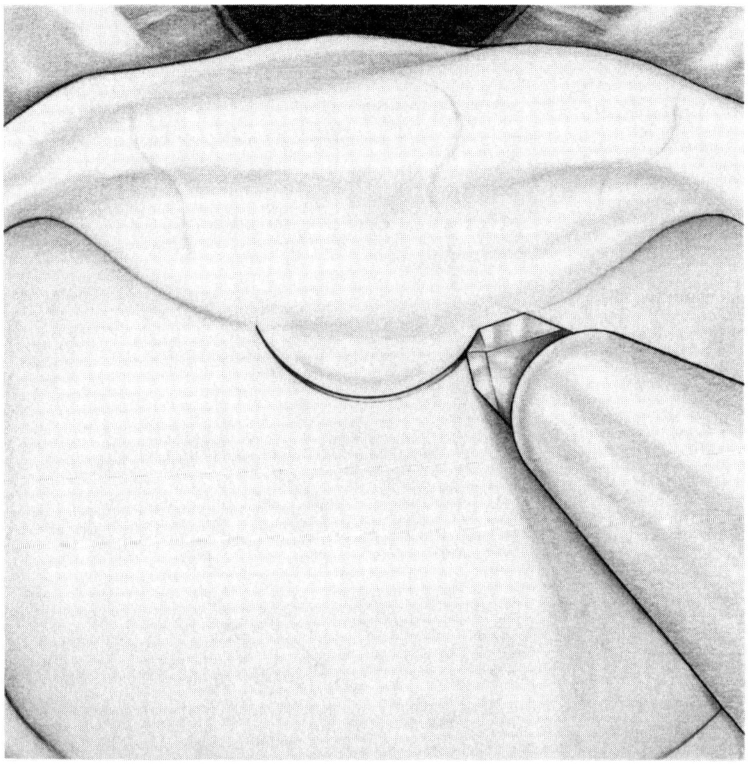

Figure 7–3

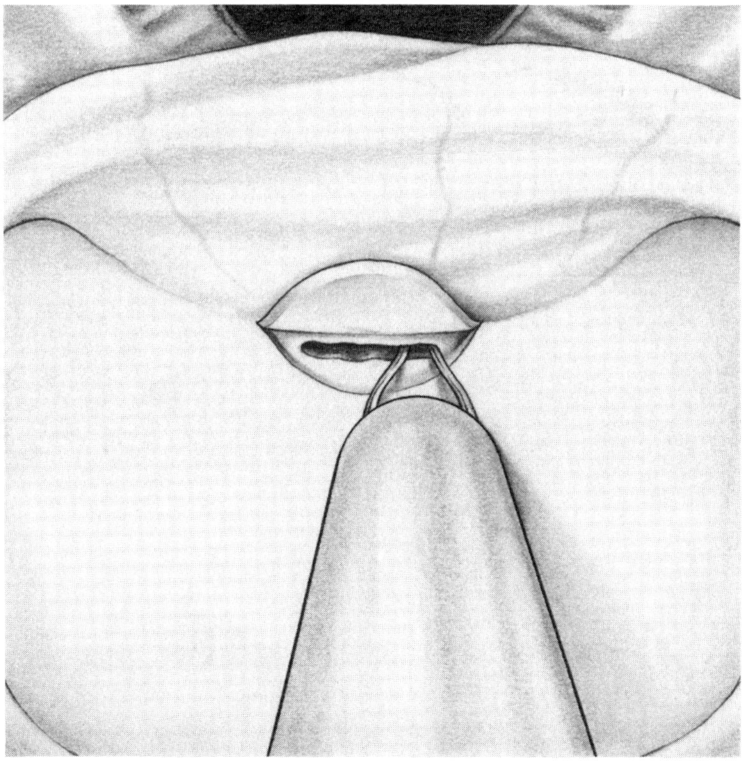

Figure 7–4

Figure 7–5. These burns produce a conical shape of the cautery entry through the sclera into the anterior chamber. Using this method, entry into the ciliary body, caused by an approach that is too posterior, or damaging the conjunctiva and Tenon's tissue by one that is too anterior both are avoided.

Figure 7–6. Once the cautery has been completed, there is little need for a protective effect of the superficial scleral lamella. A through-and-through opening is now present into the anterior chamber, and the scleral layer is excised, with the surgeon being certain that its anteriormost extension does not compromise the sclerostomy site and avoiding damage to the conjunctival–Tenon's layer during the excision. The scissors should be oriented parallel to the limbus.

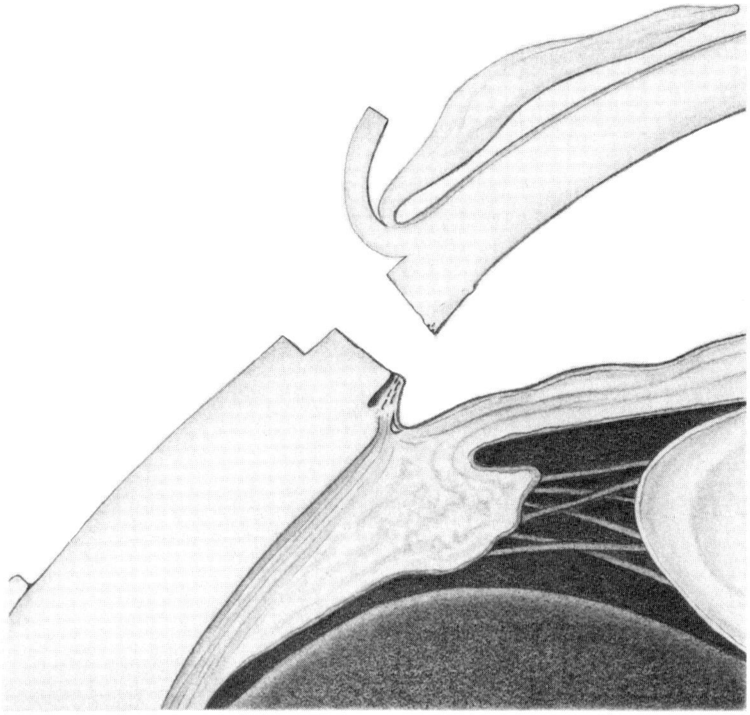

Figure 7–5

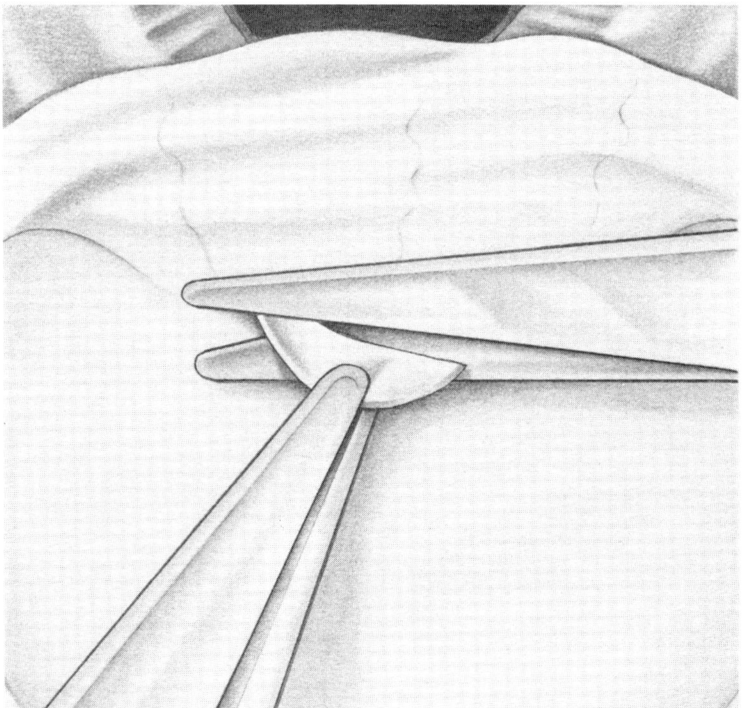

Figure 7–6

Figure 7–7. Slight pressure is placed on the posterior lip of the sclerostomy to prolapse iris into the lips of the wound. The tissue is then grasped, withdrawn, and excised to perform an iridectomy that is slightly wider than the sclerostomy opening. The technique for a two-incision iris excision also can be performed to ensure an adequately wide iridectomy (See Figs. 4–5 and 4–6).

Figure 7–8. The conjunctival-Tenon's layer is closed with a continuous running suture that apposes the tissue in two layers. An 8-0 or 9-0 Vicryl suture is appropriate for this closure.

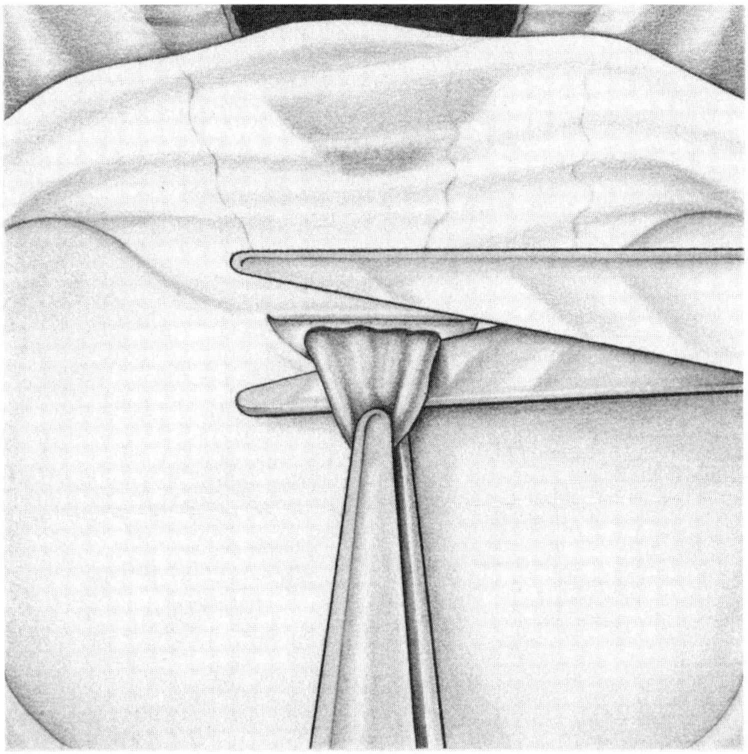

Figure 7–7

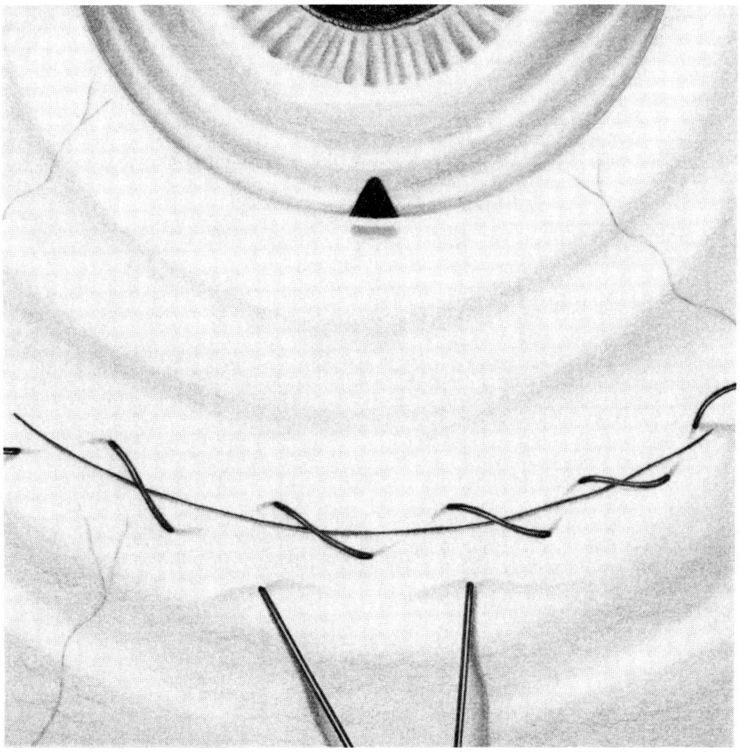

Figure 7–8

8

Cyclodialysis

Cyclodialysis is a procedure that was popular in the past but has been largely supplanted by newer microsurgical procedures. Reserved mainly for aphakic eyes, the procedure was performed internally by disinserting the ciliary body and choroid from the sclera. It is believed that aqueous moves between the anterior chamber and suprachoroidal space to keep these tissues separated, resulting in reduced aqueous secretion. One potential complication of this operation is unpredictable hypotony.

Although this procedure is performed less frequently, its basic elements are incorporated into the trabeculectomy procedure, with disinsertion behind the scleral spur, which is described in Chapter 6.

Figure 8–1. Initially, a paracentesis through clear cornea is performed. A conjunctival incision is made in a superior quadrant between the rectus muscles.

Figure 8–2. The scleral tissue is prepared with the hemostatic eraser or light cautery to control superficial bleeding. This area is located 4–6 mm from the limbus and is the site of the incision through the sclera.

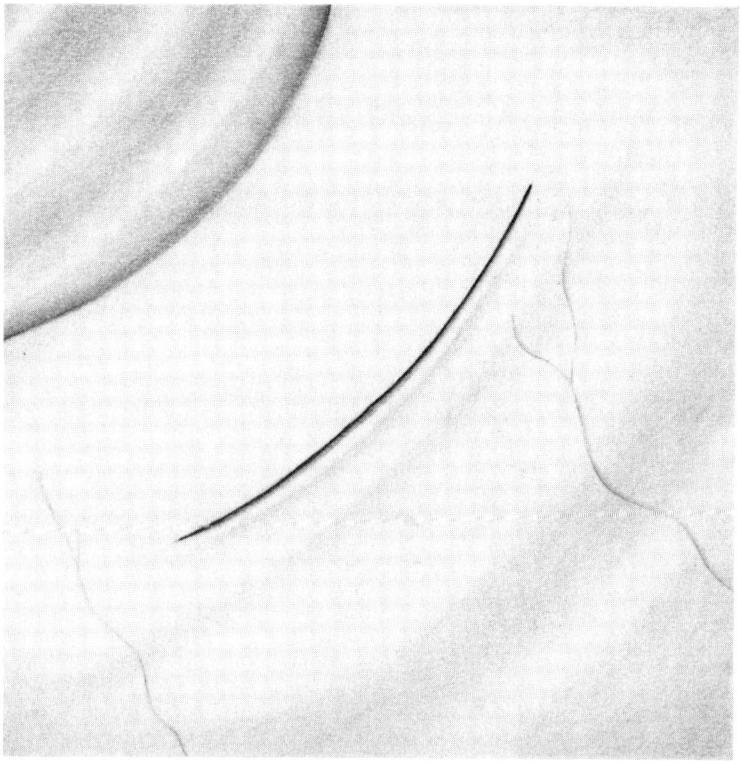

Figure 8–1

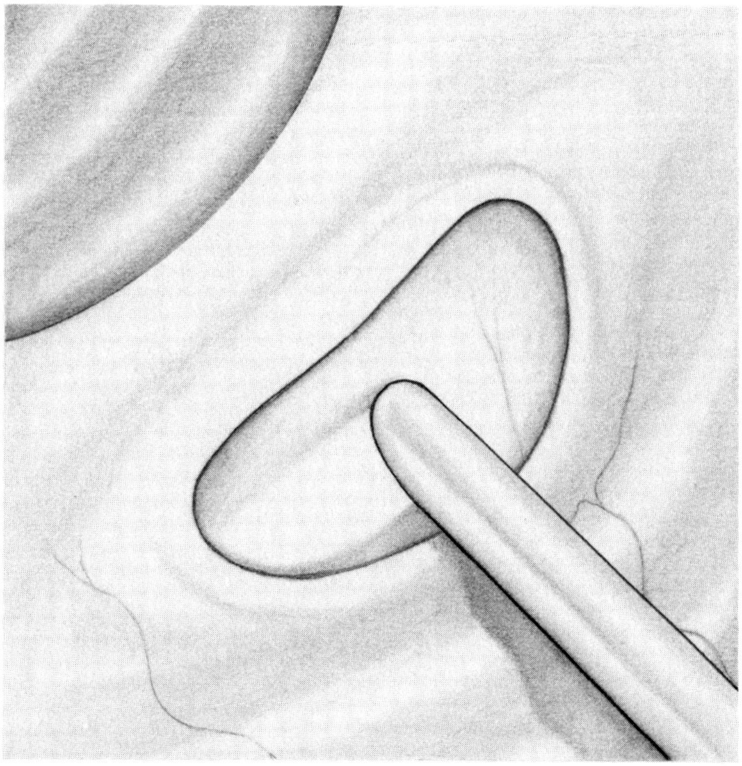

Figure 8–2

Figure 8–3. An incision perpendicular to the scleral wall is made with a rounded blade or a trifaceted diamond knife. This incision enters the suprachoroidal space. The incision is performed in a stepwise, layer-by-layer fashion to prevent precipitous damage to the underlying ciliary body and the possibility of producing a hemorrhage. The site of this scleral incision is between the superior and horizontal recti, depending on the superior quadrant selected. It is important not to move too inferior with the incision to avoid the vasculature in the horizontal meridian.

Figure 8–4. A blunt cyclodialysis spatula is introduced through the wound edges into the suprachoroidal space. The movement of the spatula is in two planes. As the spatula is advanced, upward pressure is exerted to hug the sclera and prevent entry into the ciliary body, which would result in hemorrhage and inability to achieve the desired disinsertion of the ciliary body from the sclera. The other motion of the spatula is from side to side as it is advanced and encompasses one third to one half of the extent of the intended sweep. The spatula is directed toward the extremity of the extent to be disinserted. Once the tip of the spatula is observed through the cornea, it is withdrawn slightly and then gently swept to the opposite extremity of the arc.

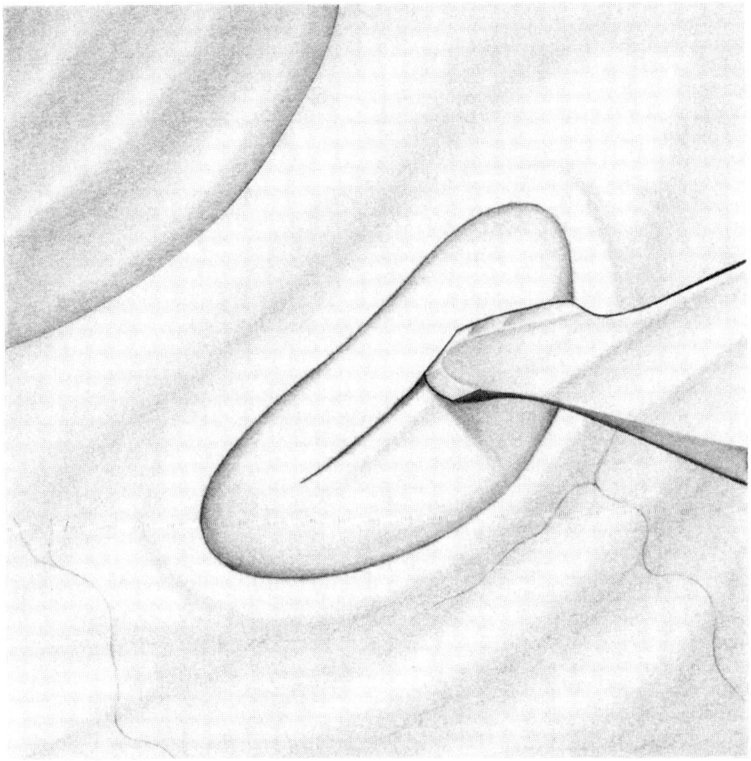

Figure 8–3

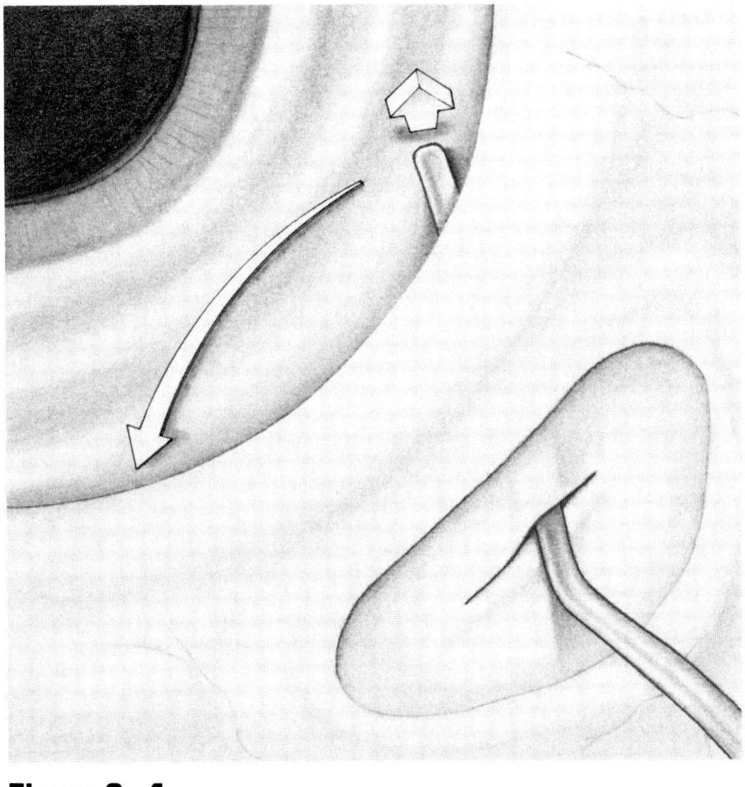

Figure 8–4

Figure 8–5. The tip of the spatula is evident in the anterior chamber. The ciliary body is disinserted at the scleral spur. The pressure on the spatula has been upward to hug the sclera and remain within the suprachoroidal space. At this point, as the spatula is swept in an arclike fashion to disinsert a larger portion of the ciliary body, a gentle ballotting action of the spatula serves to enhance the disinsertion. During this process, the cleavage plane of the spatula remains unchanged. The scleral incision can be closed with a single suture and the conjunctival incision sutured as well.

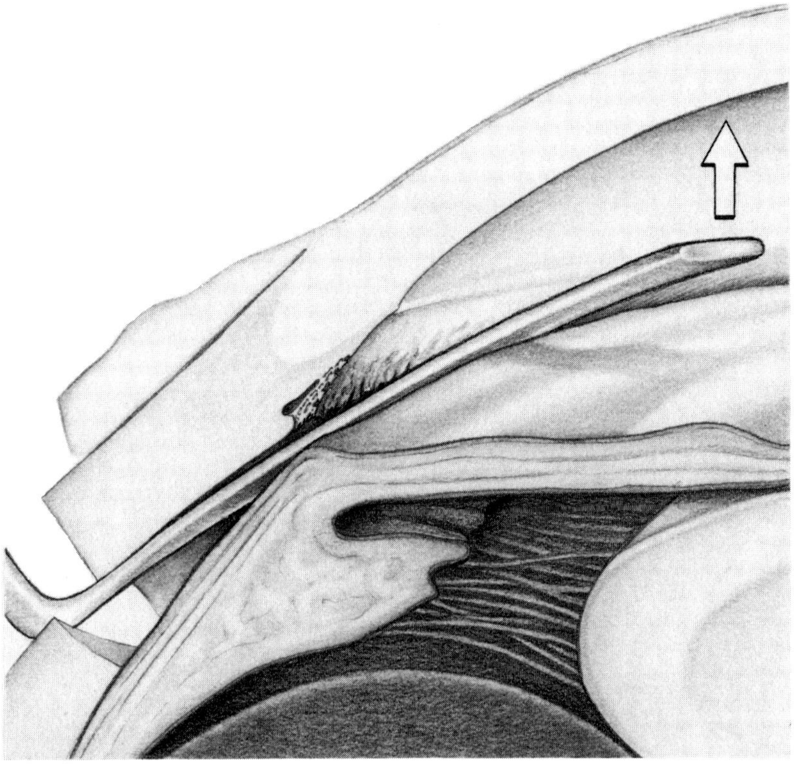

Figure 8–5

9

Surgery for Congenital Glaucoma

Currently, the primary surgery for congenital glaucoma depends on the status of the cornea. If it is clear, a goniotomy is the procedure of choice, since a direct approach to the angle and Barkan's membrane is available. If the cornea is edematous or hazy because of Haab's striae, an ab externo procedure is used. This procedure—the trabeculotomy—described by Harms and Dannheim appears to be successful if properly performed.

Figure 9–1. Visualizing the angle structures is of paramount importance in performing the goniotomy. A variety of lenses has been designed to examine the angle and to perform the goniotomy. I prefer a lens that can be secured to the globe, since it positions the eye properly for surgery and does not move during the operative procedure. There are several Worst-style lenses available for this purpose. Another feature of this lens is that irrigation is delivered through a port on the lens to eliminate air bubbles between the lens and the cornea. An incision parallel to the iris is made through clear cornea temporally to avoid operating over the nose.

Figure 9–2. A viscoelastic agent is then introduced into the anterior chamber to maintain the corneal dome and preserve good visualization of the angle structures. Formerly, this step was difficult, since the knife incision into the anterior chamber was carried across the entire chamber to the opposite angle. Using the viscoelastic agent permits a controlled incision into the anterior chamber and introduction of the goniotomy knife across a formed chamber, with little chance of damaging the iris, lens, or cornea.

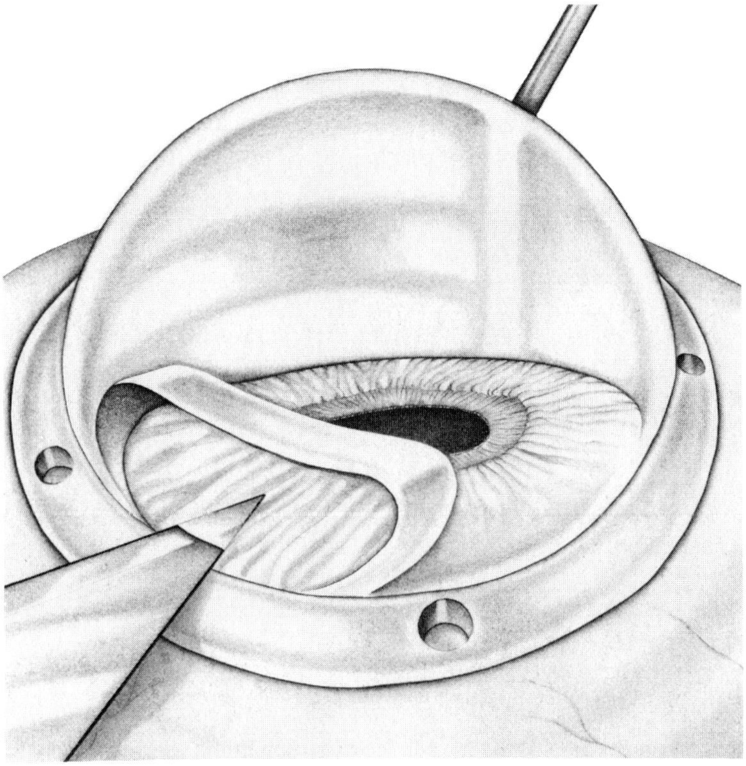

Figure 9–1

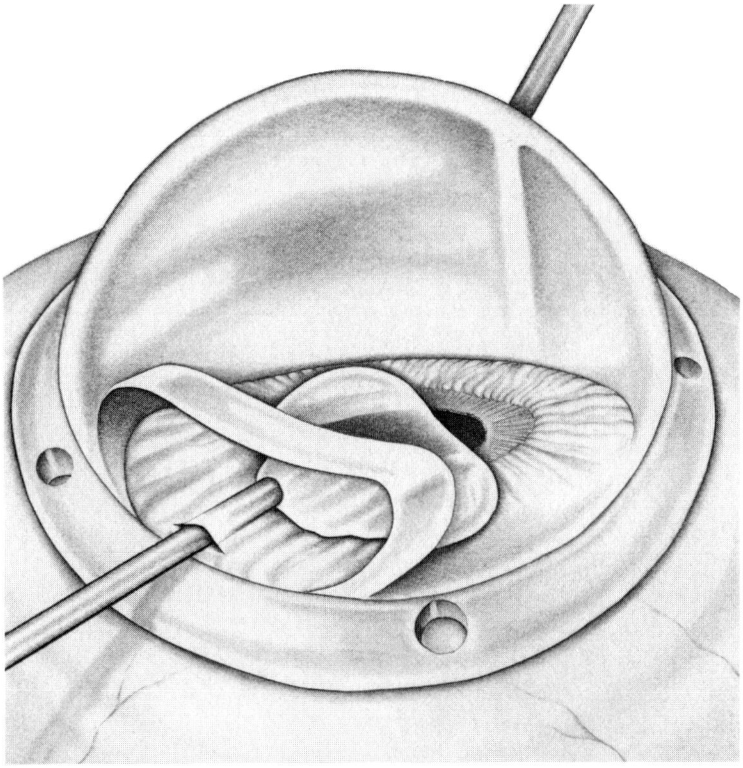

Figure 9–2

Figure 9–3. The tip of the goniotomy knife just engages Barkan's membrane and is first moved to the left (counterclockwise) and then to the right (clockwise) for approximately 4 clock hours. The angle deepens in this area as the peaking and bays of iris fall backward. It is important not to incise too deeply, since it is only necessary to remove the superficial membranous tissue, and excessive depth will cause bleeding. A benefit of the viscoelastic substance is that the width of the angle is maintained throughout the procedure, and visualization is preserved. The goniotomy knife is withdrawn, and the goniolens is removed from the surface of the globe. Since the corneal incision is small and bevelled, suturing generally is not required.

Figure 9–4. The trabeculotomy procedure approaches the angle from the exterior. Therefore, it is less precise in the anatomic removal of Barkan's membrane but, nonetheless, is an effective operation. Either a limbal or a fornix-based conjunctival flap is mobilized, depending on the surgeon's preference. A superficial scleral dissection, as described for trabeculectomy (see Chapter 6), is performed. This scleral flap, however, should be slightly thicker than the flap used for the trabeculectomy procedure. It should be at least one half or, preferably, two thirds of scleral thickness. The dissection is carried forward just to clear cornea. Under moderately high magnification, one often can note a change in color in the transition from the cornea to scleral tissue. Below this area lies Schlemm's canal, which is the important structure in this procedure. A scratchdown radial incision is performed in this area just to enter Schlemm's canal. An incision that is made too anteriorly will enter the anterior chamber through the corneal tissue, and one that is too deep will cause aqueous leakage directly from the anterior chamber.

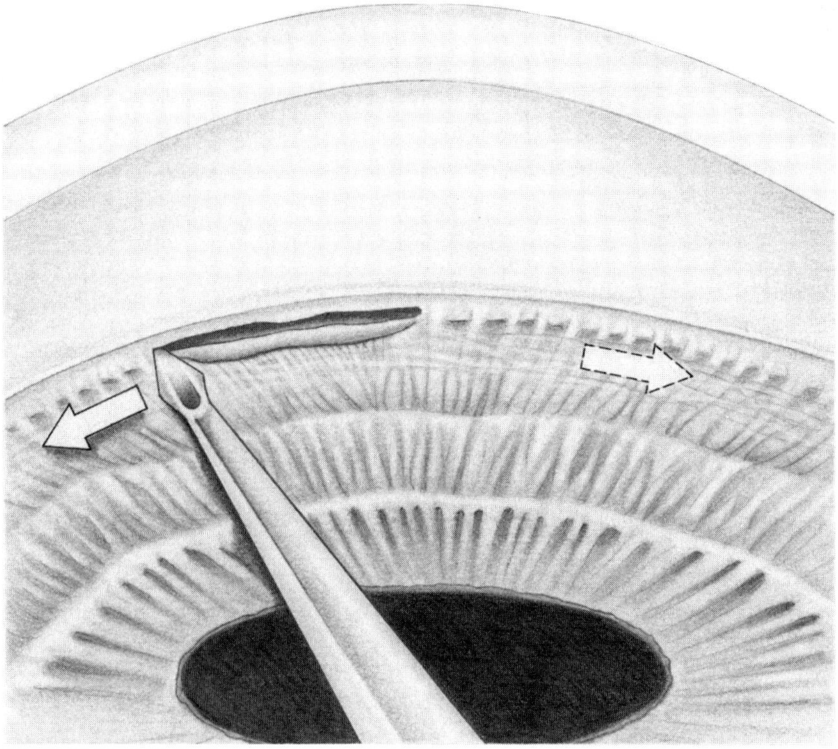

Figure 9–3

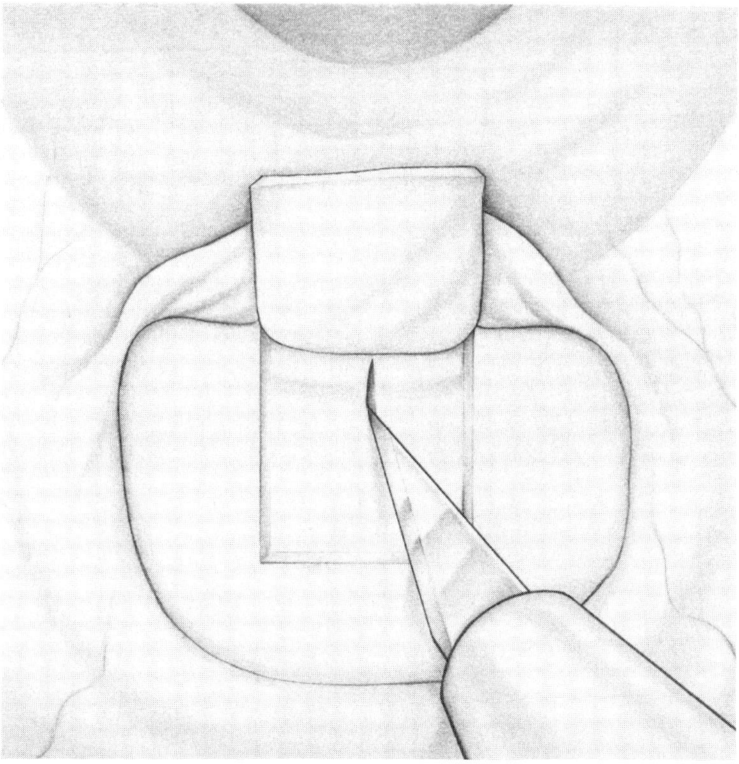

Figure 9–4

Figure 9–5. A carefully performed radial incision into Schlemm's canal is noted when aqueous percolates through the edges of the wound and saturates a fluorescein strip. However, aqueous leakage from the anterior chamber could accomplish the same effect. Everting the edges of the wound with forceps often permits the surgeon to discover if the incision is too deep or too anteriorly placed.

Figure 9–6. A Harms' trabeculotome is then introduced into the ostium of Schlemm's canal. Once again, high magnification is required to achieve the desired result. The trabeculotome is doubly wired so that the orientation of the inner wire can be monitored externally. The inner wire is introduced gently and slowly in an attempt to remain within Schlemm's canal. It is impossible to know if the trabeculotome remains in Schlemm's canal even if the initial portion of the passage has been achieved. Two points are important, however: (1) that the trabeculotome is advanced slowly and (2) that the curve of the trabeculotome is followed.

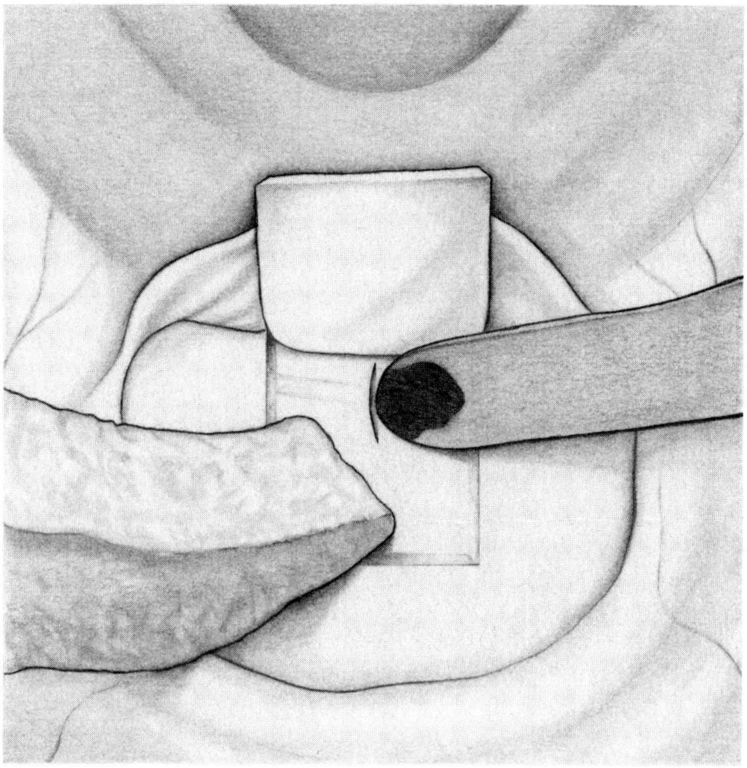

Figure 9–5

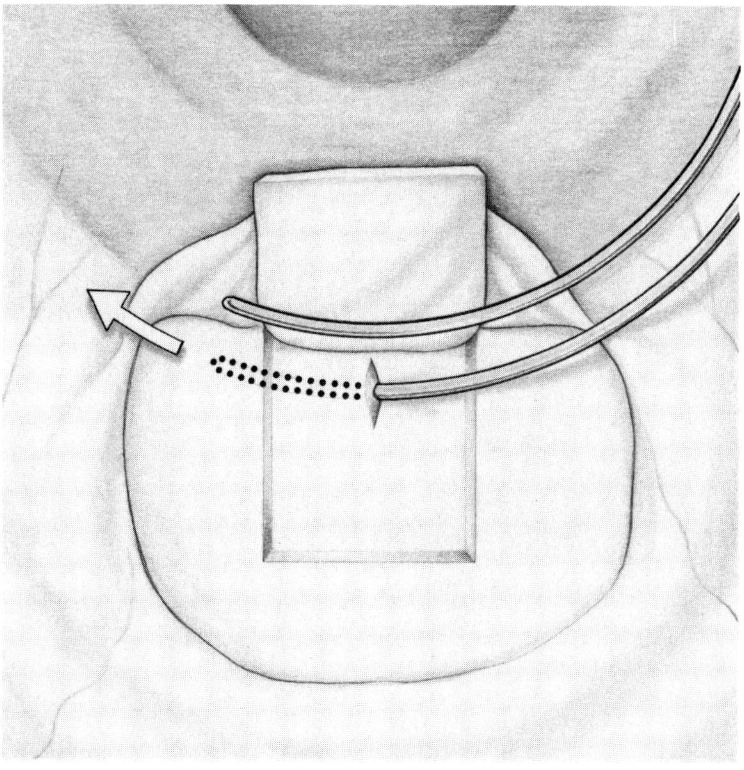

Figure 9–6

Figure 9–7. Once the length of the wire has been fully introduced, the handle is twirled in the fingers to break through the inner aspects of the angle tissue. This must be done slowly and deliberately to ensure that the trabeculotome sweeps in the angle and not posteriorly in iris substance or anteriorly to strip Descemet's membrane. Generally, the trabeculotome moves easily and without much resistance when the procedure is properly performed.

Figure 9–8. After one side has been completed, the complementary trabeculotome is introduced on the other side, and the procedure is repeated. The trabeculotome should be rotated only enough so that its length reaches the region just superior to the pupil. Too much rotation could risk damage to the lens by the tip of the trabeculotome. This means that an area of the angle between the two points of introduction of the trabeculotome, left and right, probably will remain intact and that the angle distal to this point will show destruction of Barkan's membrane.

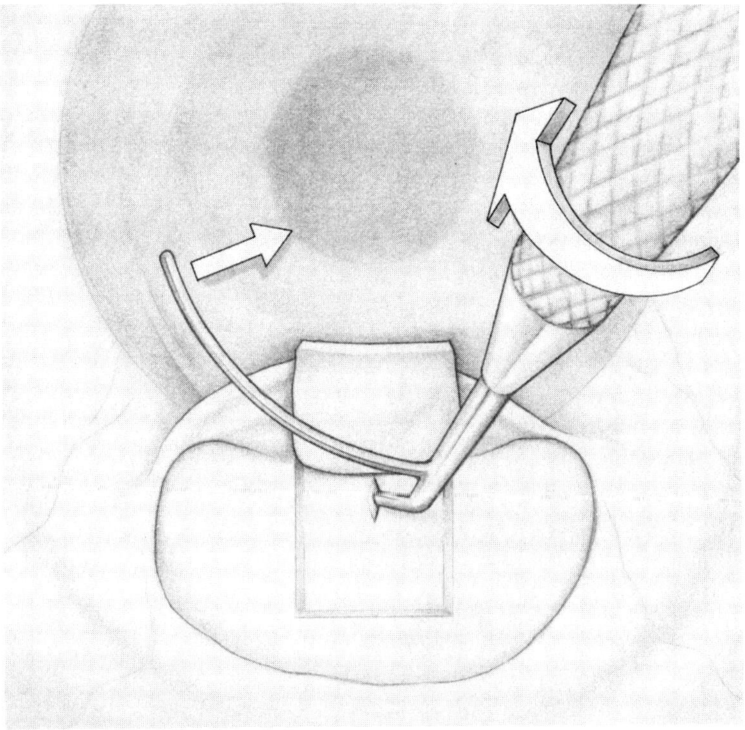

Figure 9–7

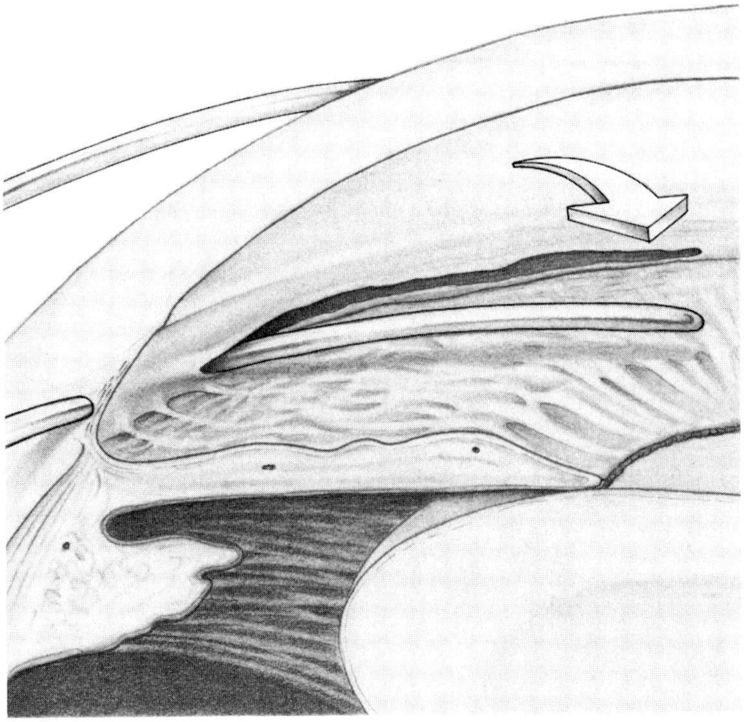

Figure 9–8

10

Surgery for Ciliary Block (Malignant) Glaucoma

Aqueous misdirection produces a type of angle-closure glaucoma that frequently can be treated medically using cycloplegic, mydriatic agents. When this regimen is unsuccessful, a surgical approach is required. A variety of techniques has been advocated to treat this condition, including lens extraction, posterior sclerotomy with incision into the vitreous before cataract extraction, perilenticular incision into the vitreous, vitreous puncture and aspiration, anterior pars plana vitrectomy, and laser therapy. My experience has been limited to cases where a modification of the technique initially described by Simmons (1972), vitreous puncture and aspiration, was used. This technique is described in greatest detail in this chapter. However, the use of vitrectomy instruments is fast supplanting this technique as the procedure of choice.

Figure 10–1. Radial incisions to the suprachoroidal space are made in the inferior quadrants about 4 mm from the limbus. These incisions serve to determine whether there is blood or fluid present, which would contradict the diagnosis of malignant or ciliary block glaucoma produced by aqueous misdirection. If there is no blood or fluid present, the nasal incision is closed. A paracentesis incision is made through clear cornea for air injection, which will be performed near the end of the procedure.

Figure 10–2. The mechanism causing angle closure is the posterior misdirection of aqueous flow, which displaces the vitreous forward, blocking the anterior outflow channels. The anterior chamber is shallow, but miotics only worsen the condition.

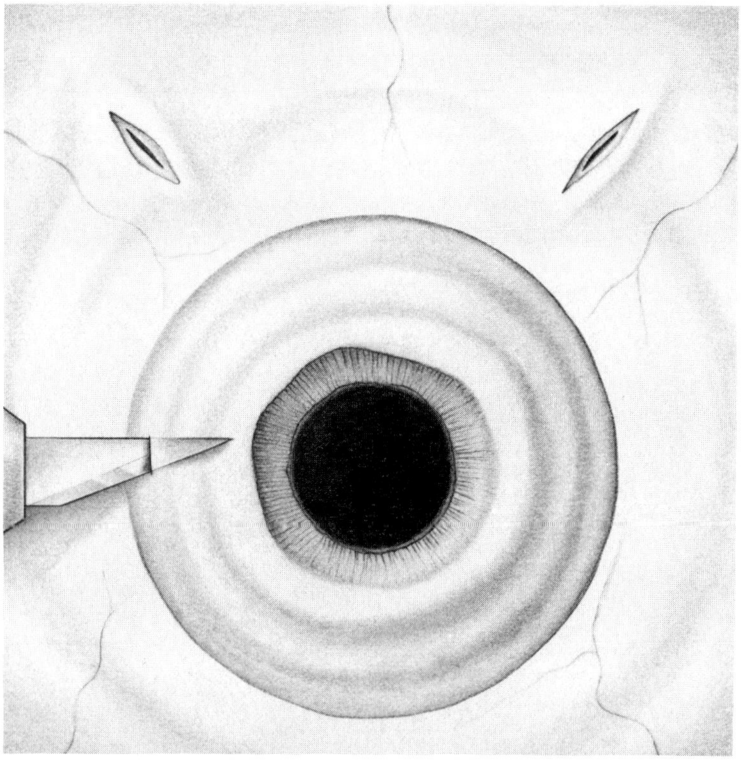

Figure 10–1

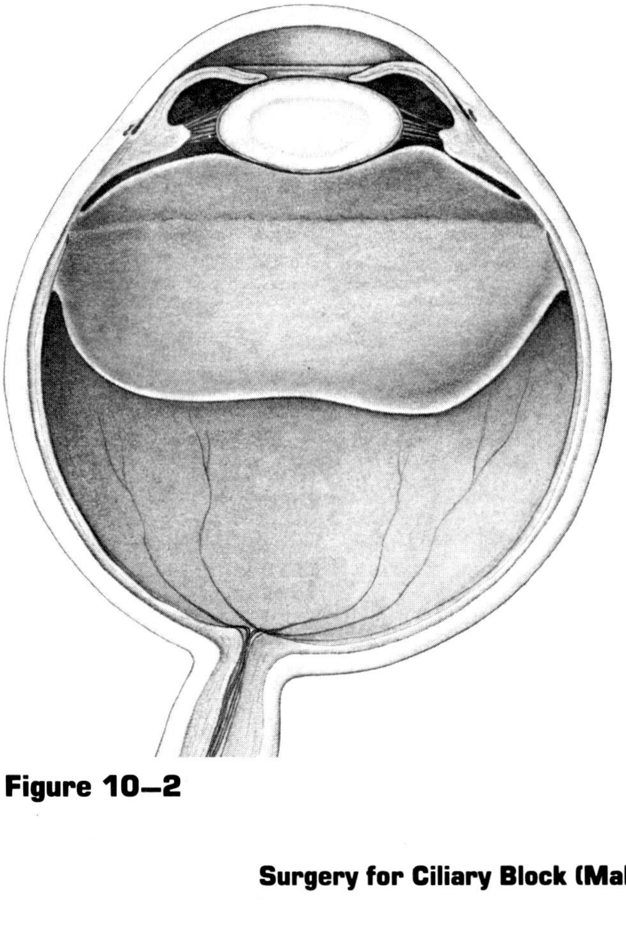

Figure 10–2

Figure 10–3. The inferotemporal incision is surrounded with diathermy. This site is used for the passage of an MVR blade through the pars plana, the anteriorly placed vitreous, and the posteriorly pooled aqueous. The MVR blade is directed toward the optic nerve that angles away from the periphery of the lens. It is important to use a sharp blade to form a tract from the incision through the posterior structures.

Figure 10–4. A hemostat is placed 12 mm from the tip of an 18-gauge needle. This precaution ensures control of the depth of penetration of the needle into the eye to prevent inadvertent retinal damage. Once the needle has been passed to the full 12 mm length, the tip of the needle is moved from side to side to widen the previously formed tract. Often, during this step, posteriorly pooled aqueous will pass around the shaft of the needle and exit through the wound. About 1.5 mm of fluid is then withdrawn into the syringe.

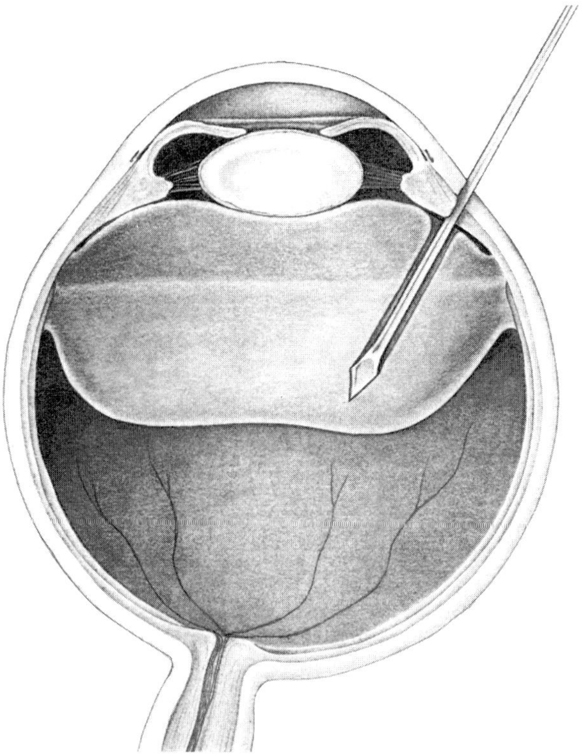

Figure 10–3

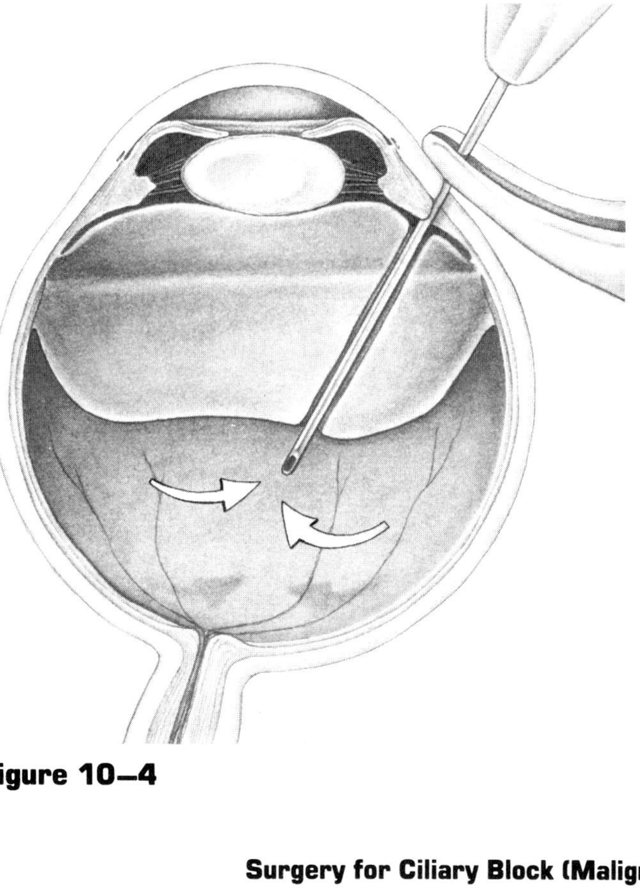

Figure 10–4

Figure 10–5. When this situation occurs in the aphakic eye, a limbal approach is used instead of the incision's being made through the pars plana. The MVR blade enters the vitreous through the pupil, and the 18-gauge needle is introduced in a similar manner. This procedure is somewhat easier, since the lens is no longer an impediment to visualization.

Figure 10–6. The eye is now soft because of the removal of the posteriorly pooled aqueous. The plane of the iris will flatten and the chamber deepen because there is no posterior pressure forcing the contents anteriorly. A large air bubble is injected through the previously prepared paracentesis site to deepen the anterior chamber excessively. The pupil is then dilated with atropine to tighten the zonular fibers and maintain the lens in a posterior orientation.

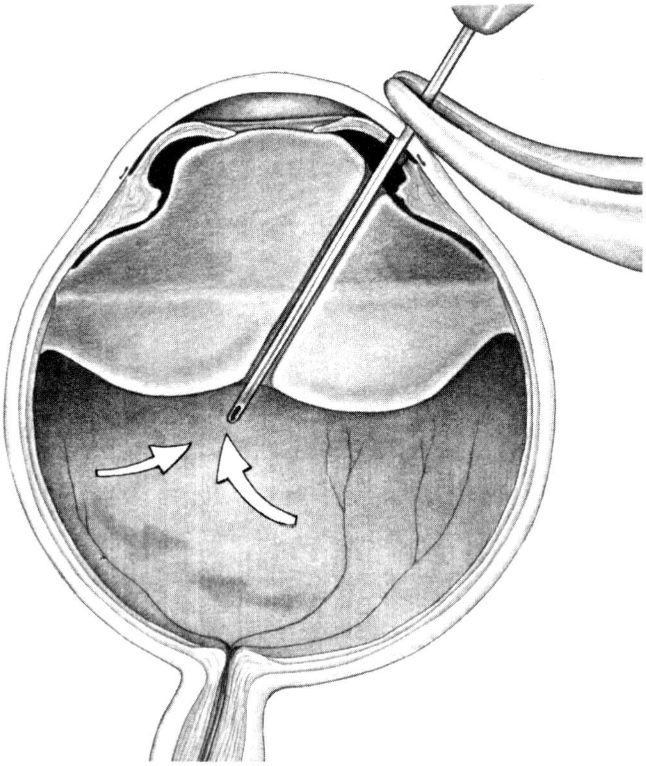

Figure 10–5

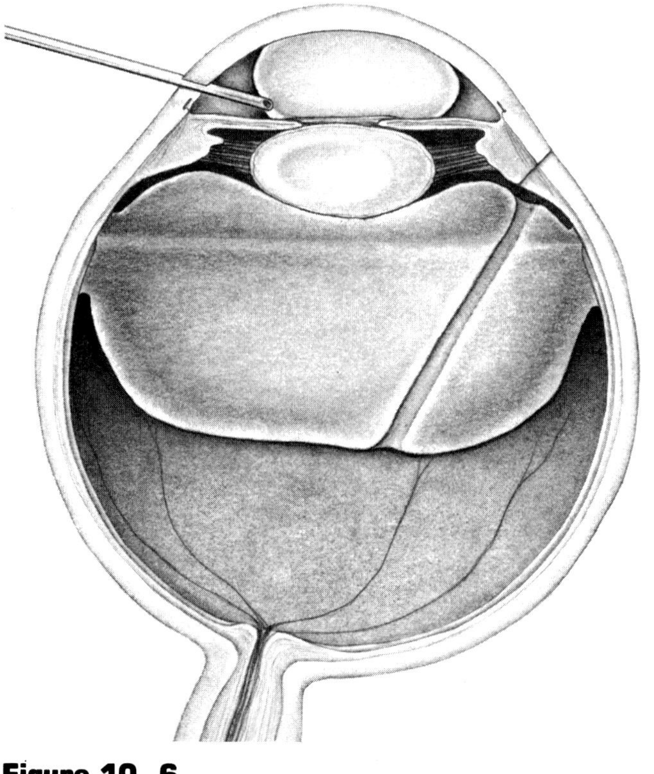

Figure 10–6

Figure 10–7. In recent years, automated vitrectomy units have been applied in instances where so-called ciliary block after intraocular lens (IOL) procedures have been encountered. So, too, they can be applied in those conditions resulting in malignant glaucoma or ciliary block glaucoma. A pars plana approach is used to introduce the vitrectomy instrument, and a core vitrectomy is performed until the pocket of aqueous is reached. (A, aqueous; V, vitreous.)

Figure 10–8. This tunnel creates a communication between the posteriorly pooled aqueous and an anterior approach. The same effect is created as described in the automated vitrectomy procedure. (A, aqueous.)

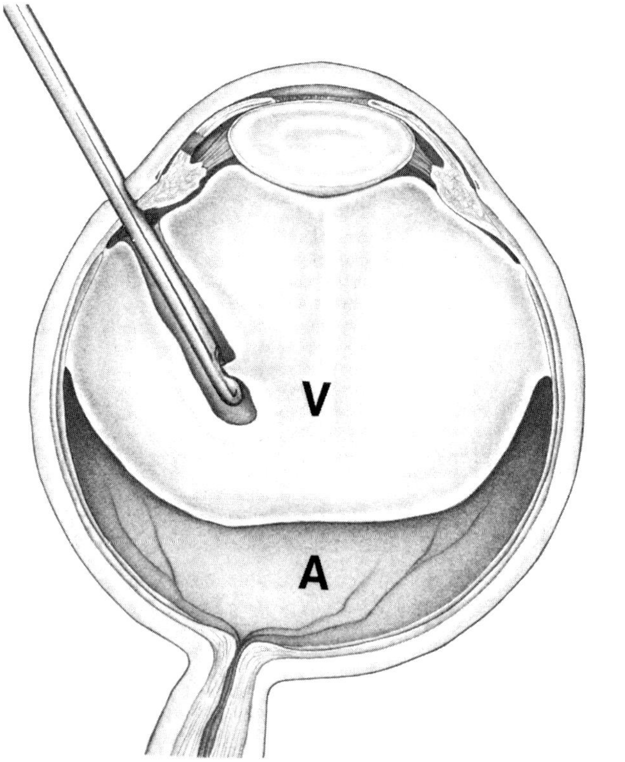

Figure 10–7

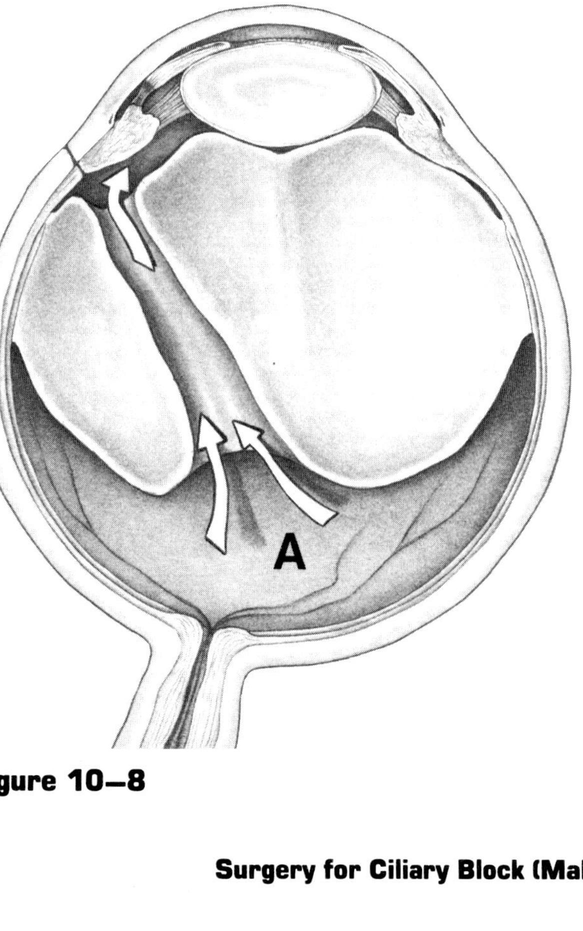

Figure 10–8

Figure 10–9. At the completion of the procedure, an air bubble is placed in the anterior chamber. The lens is shifted in a posterior position, with the addition of atropine-like drugs, and the anterior segment relationships are normalized with a cessation of the mechanism, producing the aqueous misdirection.

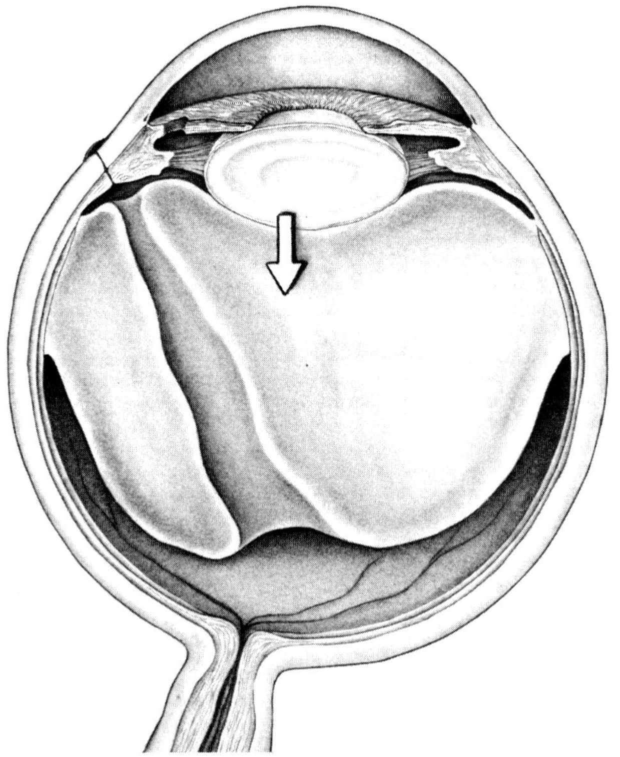

Figure 10–9

11

Surgery for Glaucoma, Cataract, and Intraocular Lens Implantation

As our population ages, the prevalence of cataract and glaucoma occurring concomitantly has increased. In eyes that require maximally tolerated medical treatment or have had previous laser trabeculoplasty or patients in whom medical treatment is not optimal, a combined surgical procedure should be performed.

Figure 11–1. A fornix-based conjunctival flap is prepared, with the surgeon being certain that it is freely mobile so that it can be drawn securely over the incision at the completion of the procedure. Bipolar cautery is applied to the sclera to control bleeding from superficial vessels and create a clean surface. A rectangular scleral flap is then outlined, and two vertically grooved, partial-thickness (50%–75%) incisions are made at the posterior limbus.

Figure 11–2. A lamellar scleral flap of about one-third to one-half thickness is dissected toward the limbus and continued until the top of the dissection blade can be viewed through clear cornea. This ensures a sufficient anterior exposure for removing the corneoscleral tissue later in the procedure.

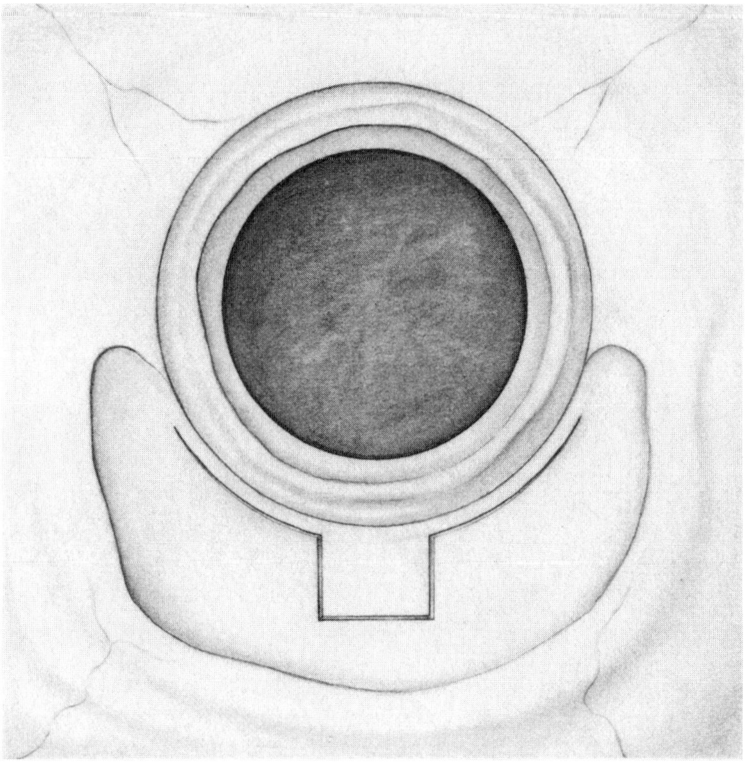

Figure 11–1

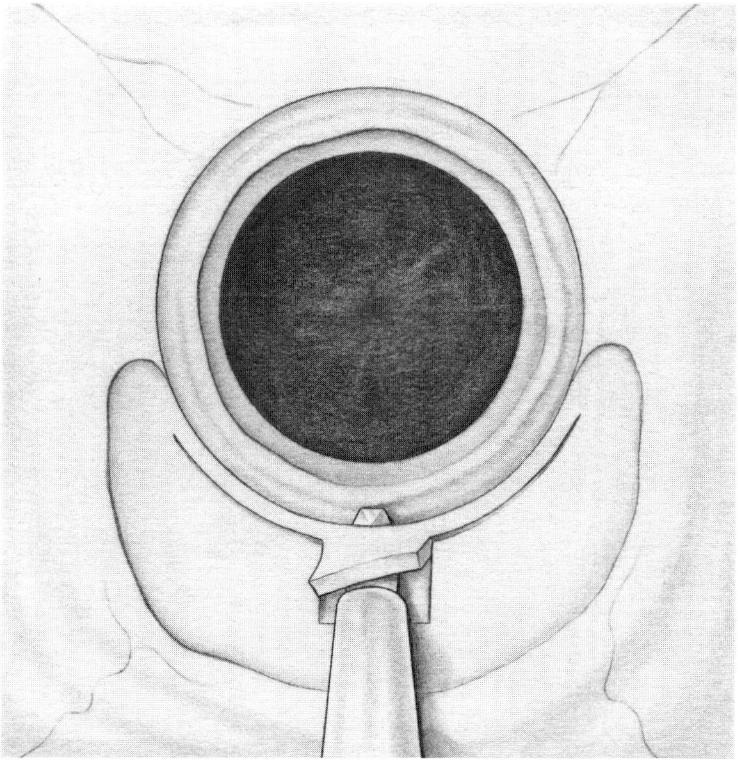

Figure 11–2

Figure 11–3. The anterior chamber is entered anteriorly at the base of the superficial scleral dissection. Healon is injected into the anterior chamber to maintain the corneal dome, widen the pupil, and coat the tissues lining the anterior chamber.

Figure 11–4. Should the pupil dilate poorly, a peripheral iridectomy and radial sphincterotomy will create an adequate opening so that an anterior capsulotomy can be performed. If the pupil is extremely miotic, synechiolysis and inferior sphincterotomy also are performed at this time.

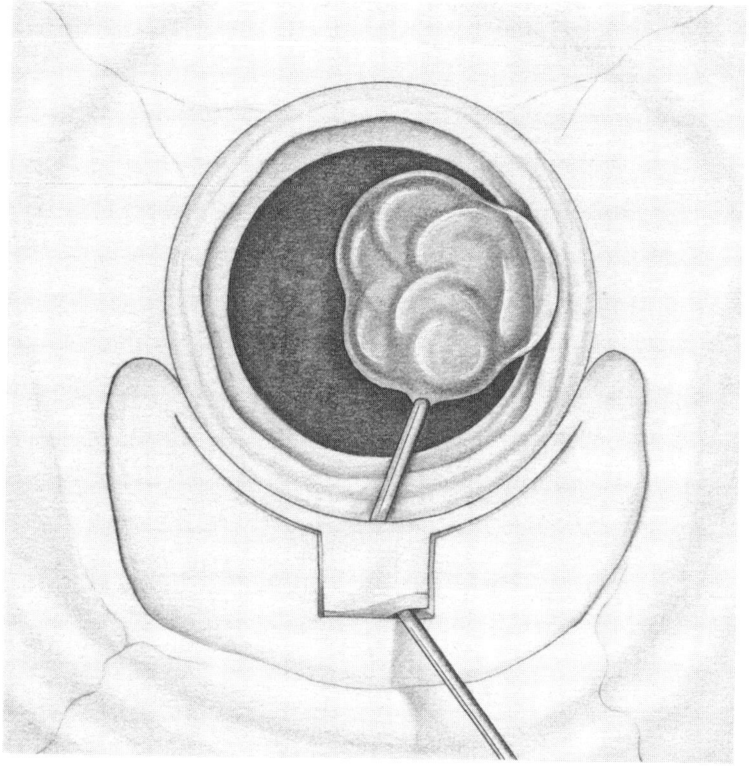

Figure 11–3

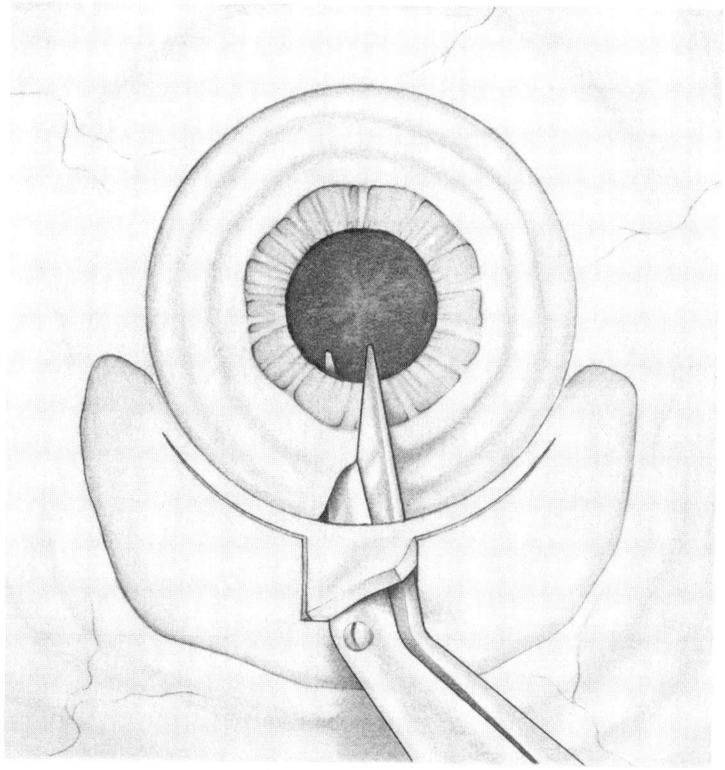

Figure 11–4

Figure 11–5. The anterior capsulectomy is performed in an anterior chamber filled with sodium hyaluronate using a bent 25-gauge needle without irrigation. If the conventional beer-can-opener capsulotomy is used, many small adjoining punctures are made in the anterior capsule so that a properly sized, well-proportioned capsulotomy is achieved. Alternatively, a slit capsulotomy for the envelope technique, as described in Chapter 12, can be performed.

Figure 11–6. The corneoscleral incision is completed with scissors for the full extent of the previously made grooved incision. The scissors are introduced parallel to the plane of the iris to create a biplaned incision.

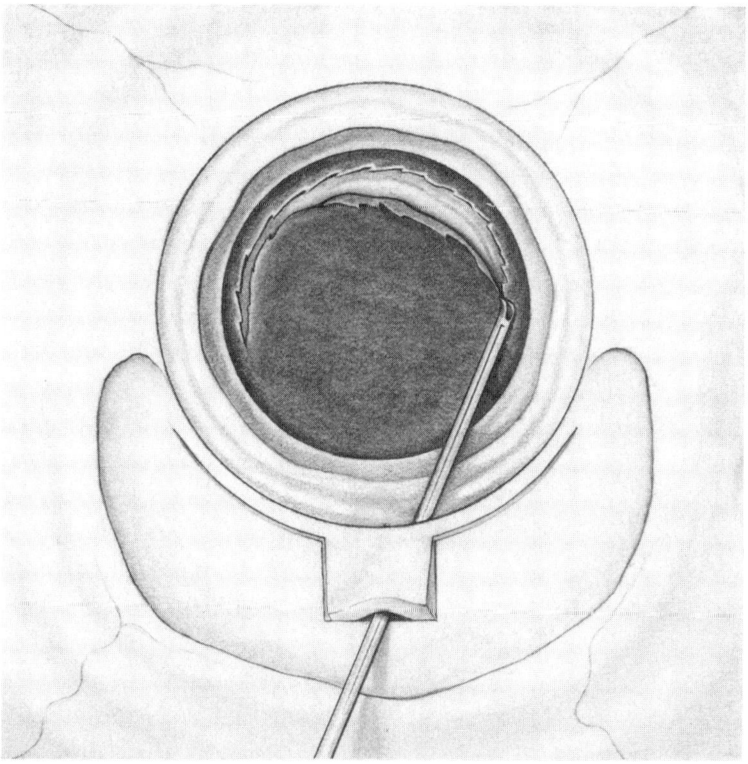

Figure 11–5

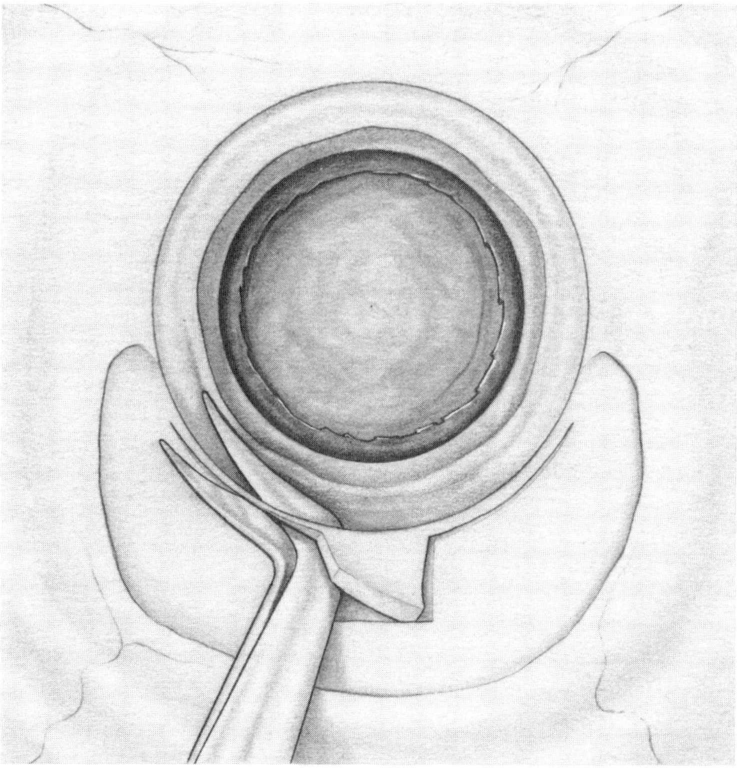

Figure 11–6

Figure 11–7. A scleral punch is introduced to abut as far into the angle as possible. The punches should remove as much tissue within the confines of the superficial dissection but should remain within this area.

Figure 11–8. A cross-sectional representation shows that, ideally, the deeper layer of the sclera is removed to the area of the insertion of the ciliary muscle at the scleral spur. In addition, a section of corneal tissue is removed.

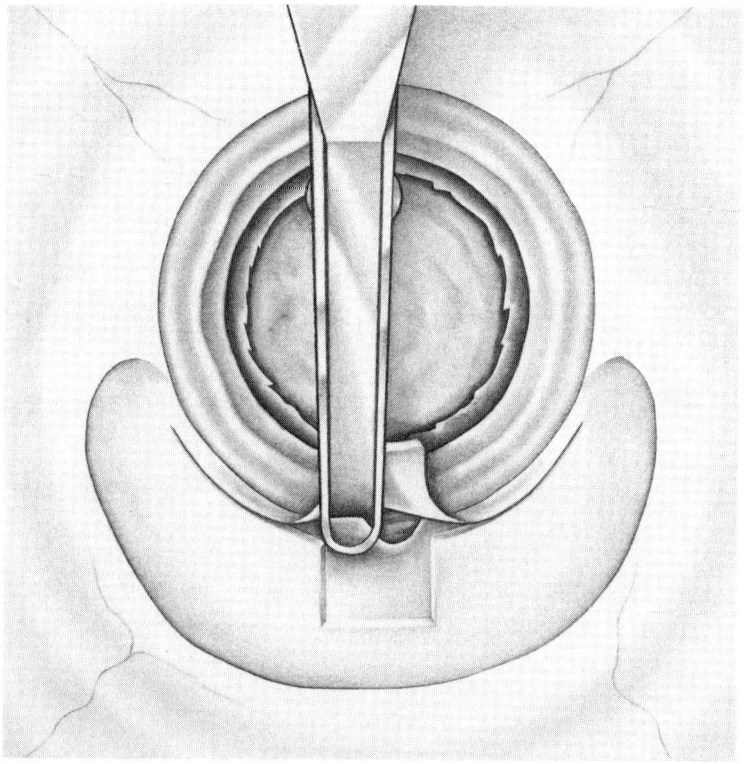

Figure 11–7

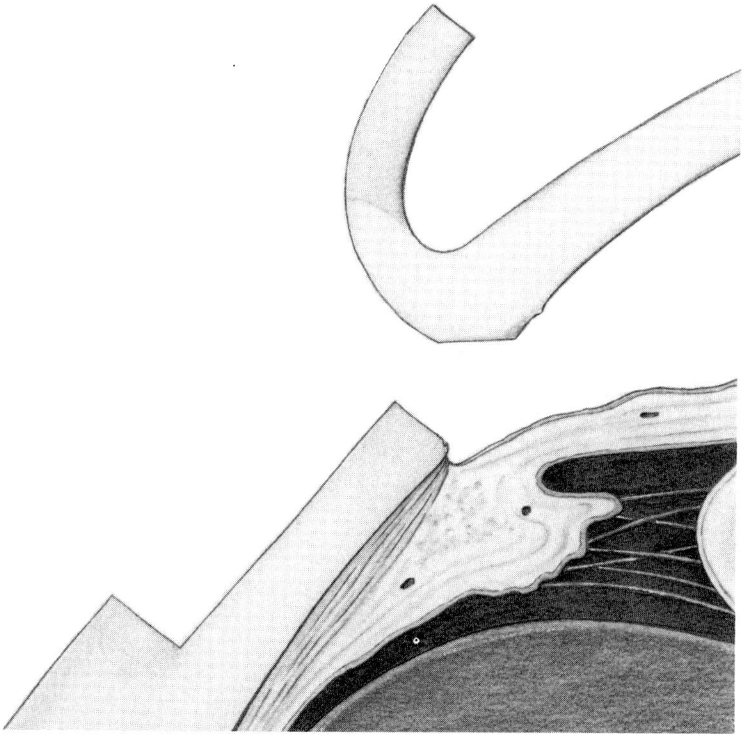

Figure 11–8

Figure 11–9. I prefer to perform the trabeculectomy portion of the procedure while the nucleus is in situ to prevent potential damage to the posterior capsule. Nucleus removal is now performed, using the surgeon's favorite technique. For nucleus expression, gentle pressure placed just within the limbus and directed posteriorly toward the optic nerve will tilt the superior pole out of the capsular bag. Gentle pressure at the superior scleral lip permits the dislodged superior pole to leave the eye in a controlled fashion.

Figure 11–10. Sutures are placed to close the peripheral portions of the cataract incision, since there is no longer a reason to maintain a wide incisional opening. Peripheral wound closure allows irrigation aspiration to be performed in a somewhat more closed system, thereby reducing anterior chamber fluid fluctuations. The degree of closure is dictated by the size of the optic of the IOL to be inserted. The position of the sutures should permit adequate space for IOL insertion for those with larger-sized optics. The posterior capsule can be polished or vacuumed at this time.

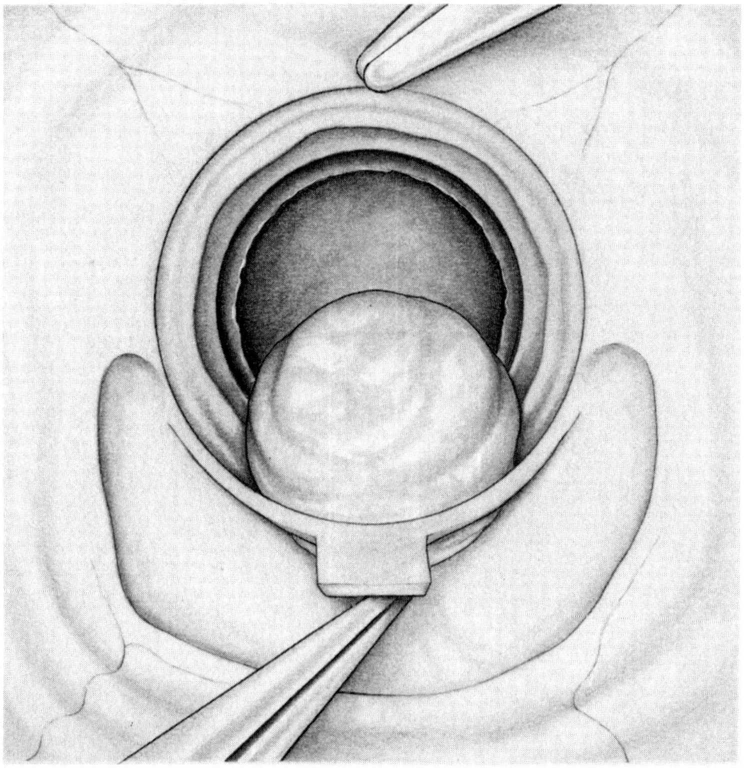

Figure 11–9

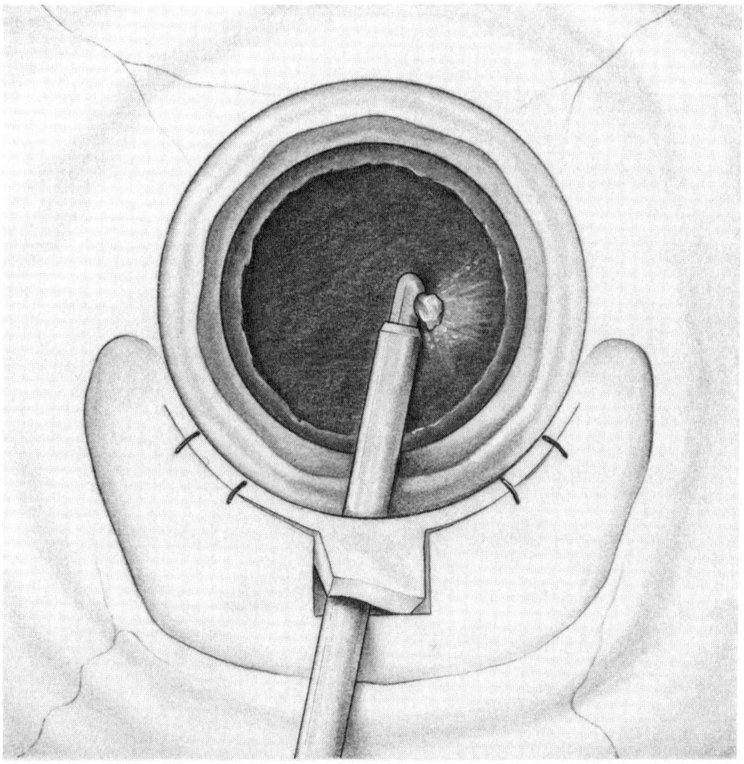

Figure 11–10

Figure 11–11. The anterior chamber is filled with a viscoelastic agent. Adequate introduction of the viscoelastic substance is judged by the slight outward rolling of the edge of the capsulotomy. The IOL optic is grasped securely to ensure a controlled introduction of the distal haptic into the capsular bag. When the envelope technique is used, the bag is filled with a viscoelastic material, and the IOL is inserted within the envelope of the capsular bag.

Figure 11–12. It is my personal preference to insert the IOL into the bag in three steps. The first, introducing the inferior or distal loop, has already been accomplished. The second step is placing the optic within the capsular bag. The superior loop is manipulated to rotate the optic into its correct position.

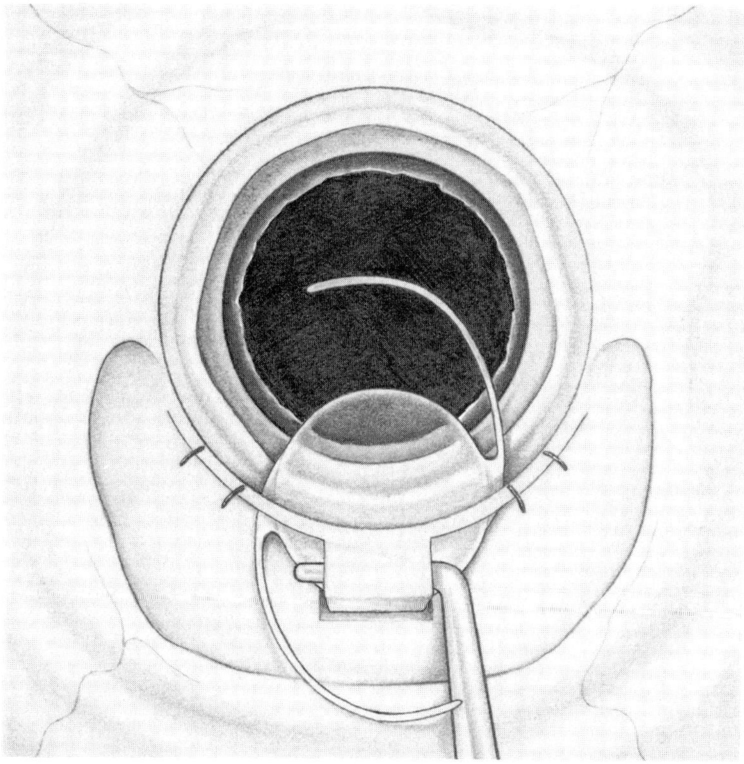

Figure 11–11

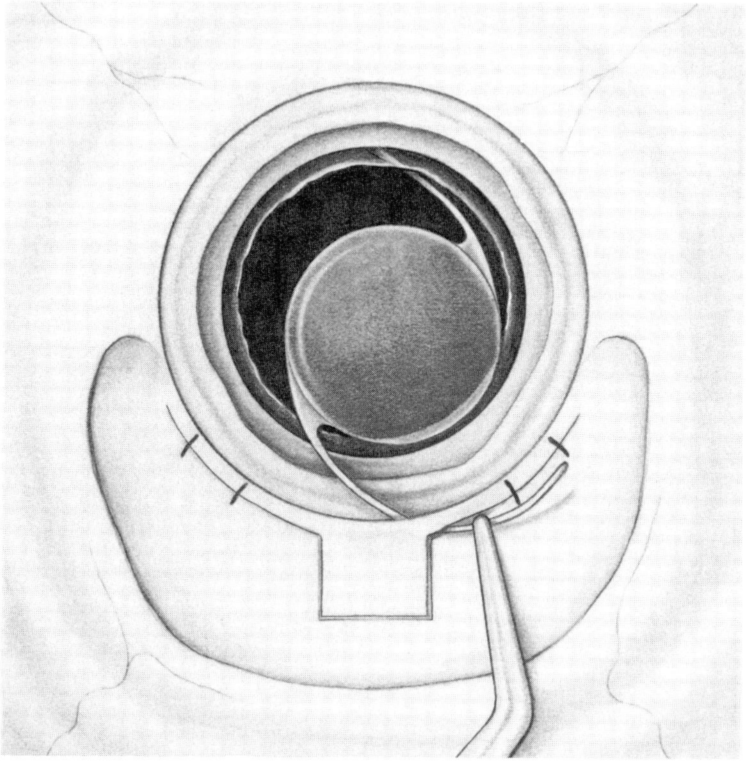

Figure 11–12

Figure 11–13. The final step of this three-step method is to place the superior or proximal haptic into the capsular bag. Two techniques can be used. In the first, the superior haptic is grasped with a Kelman–McPherson or Gaskin forceps, and the superior loop is pushed inferiorly so that the loop flexes and can be placed beneath the superior portion of the capsular bag. An alternative method is to position a Lester hook at the junction of the loop and haptic and rotate the superior loop into the capsular bag. With a one-piece PMMA lens, there is no need to rotate the IOL further, since it will center and remain in a stable position.

Figure 11–14. A peripheral iridectomy is performed at this time, if it has not been done already. The iridectomy should be as wide as the internal sclerostomy opening. This precaution will prevent synechias to the edges of the sclerostomy that ultimately can seal off the filtration site.

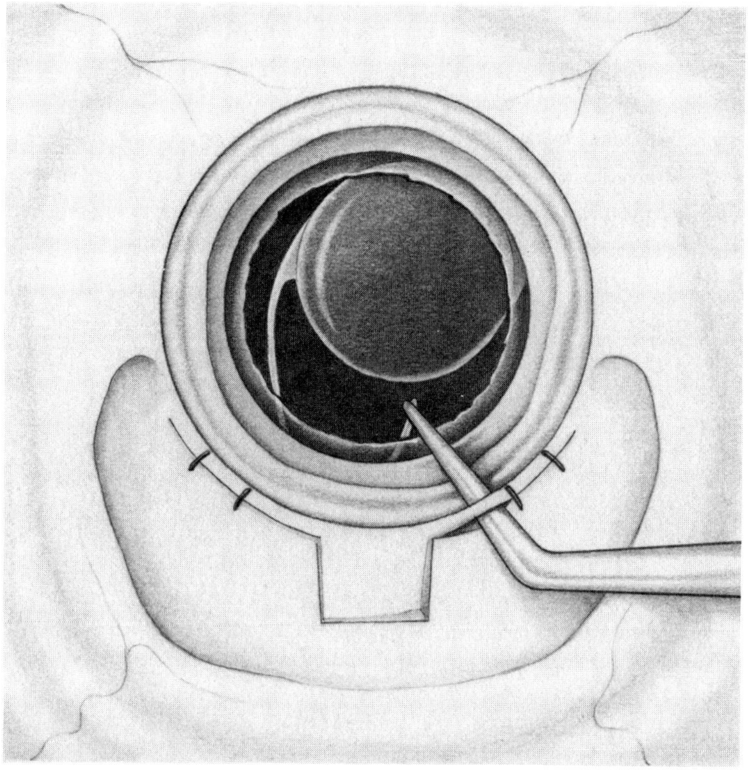

Figure 11–13

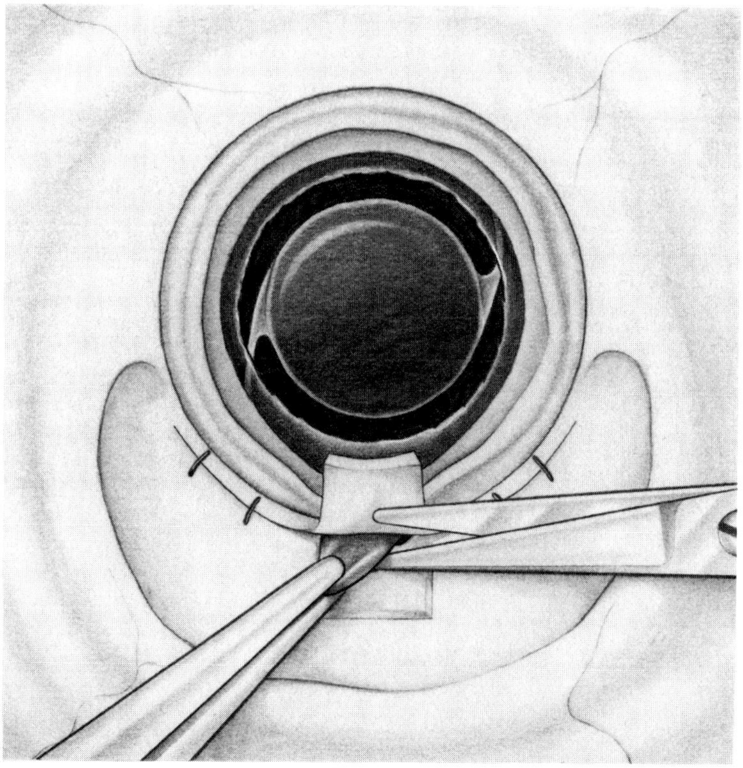

Figure 11–14

Figure 11–15. The viscoelastic material is removed by aspirating it from the anterior chamber. Pressure on the optic with the irrigation and aspiration (I&A) tip directed posteriorly often will release viscoelastic material that is sequestered in the fornices of the capsular bag. Sutures are placed at the junction of the circumferential cataract incision and the vertically placed incisions of the scleral flap. In addition, the superior corners of the superficial scleral dissection are sutured with enough tension just to appose the edges of the tissues. Sutures placed too tightly will prevent adequate filtration.

Figure 11–16. Although it is not absolutely necessary to close a full iris coloboma, one may appose the pillars of the iris by placing a suture at the iris collarette. Since this is an intracameral suture, 10-0 polypropylene suture material should be used. The suture should not be tied too tightly, since it may tear through the tissue. The conjunctival flap is brought down to cover the scleral dissection and cataract incision. The ends of the conjunctival flap are secured with Vicryl suture to keep the conjunctiva in position for several days before it can stick into its proper position by itself.

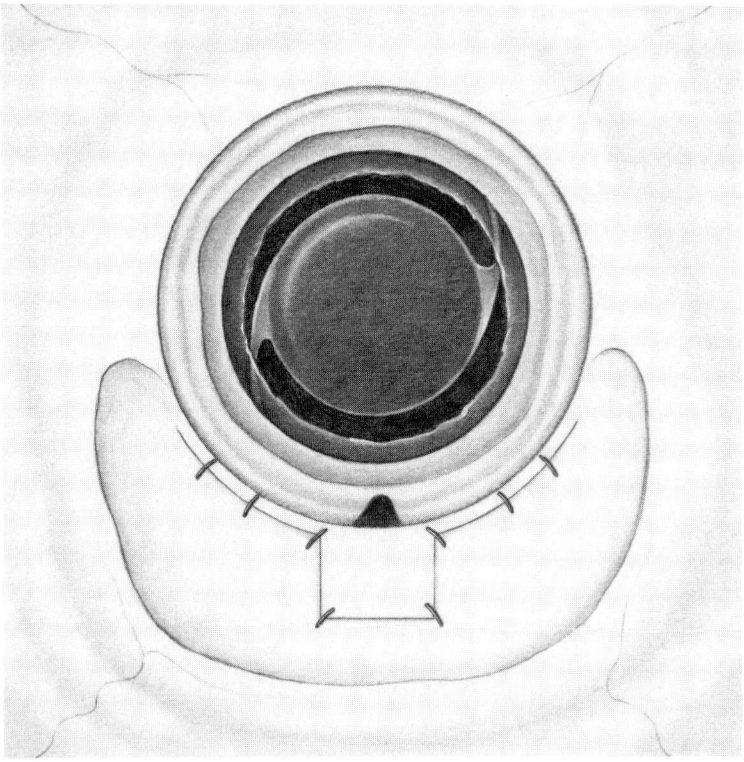

Figure 11–15

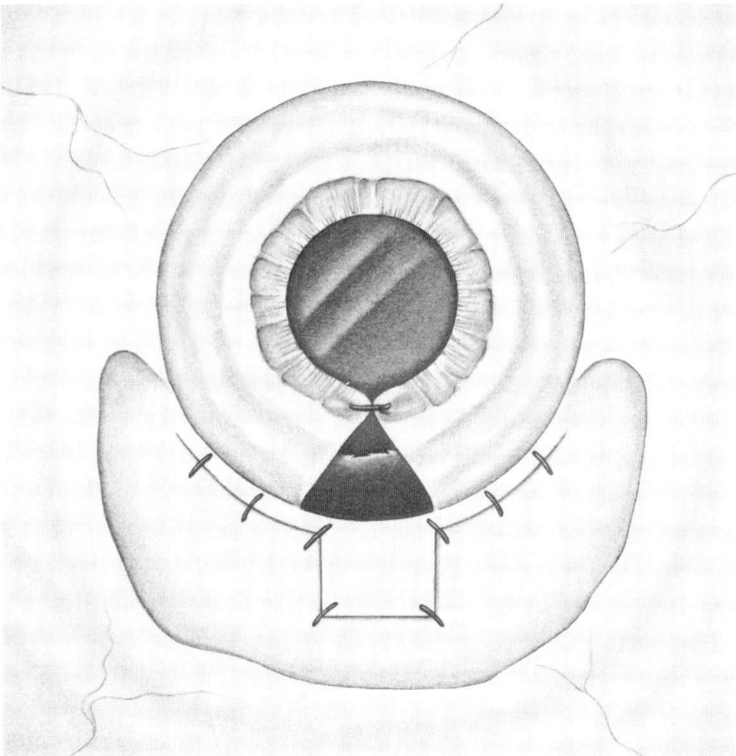

Figure 11–16

Figure 11–17. An alternate to the procedure just described is to perform the cataract—IOL and filtration procedures through distinct incisions. After preparing a limbal-based conjunctival–Tenon's flap, a superficial scleral dissection is performed. The cataract incision is then made in clear cornea.

Figure 11–18. The steps of the cataract–IOL surgery have been described previously. Once this portion of the procedure has been completed, an iridectomy is performed. The deep scleral trabeculectomy specimen is excised.

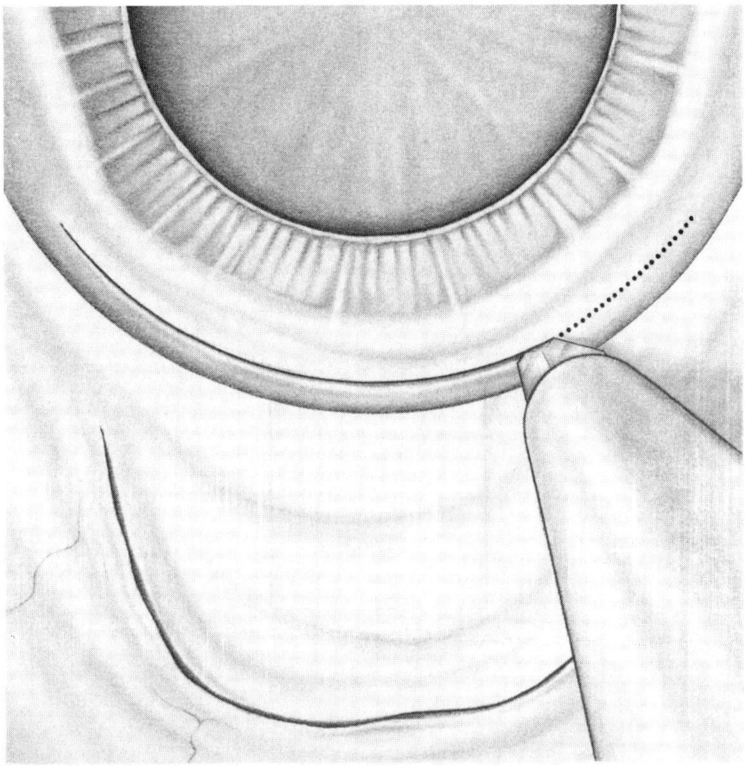

Figure 11–17

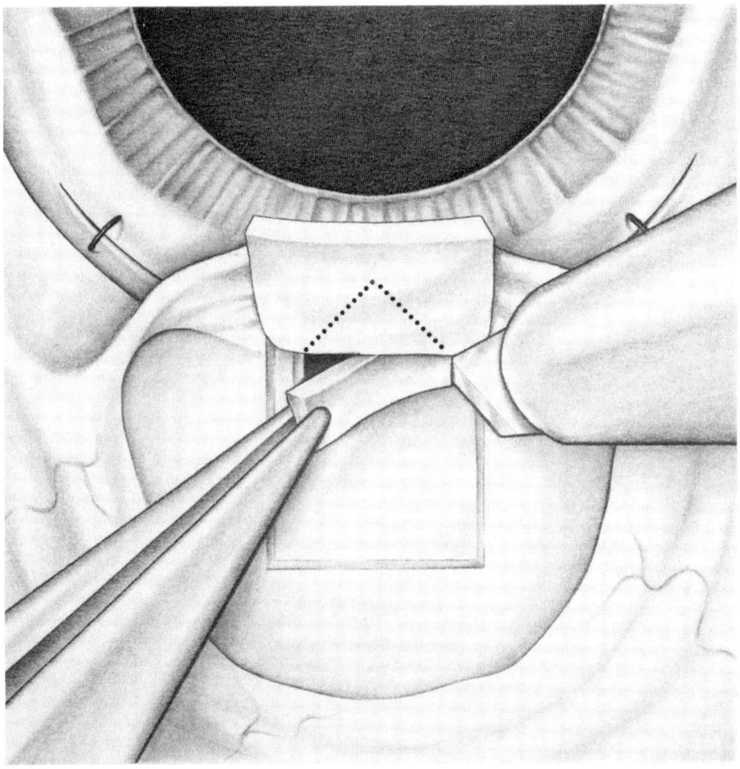

Figure 11–18

Figure 11–19. The scleral flap is closed at its corners with 10-0 nylon suture. The conjunctival–Tenon's flap is sutured with a continuous running 8-0 or 9-0 Vicryl suture. This cross-sectional view illustrates the superficial scleral dissection, the area of excised trabeculum, a peripheral iridectomy, the corneal cataract incision, and the IOL within the capsular bag.

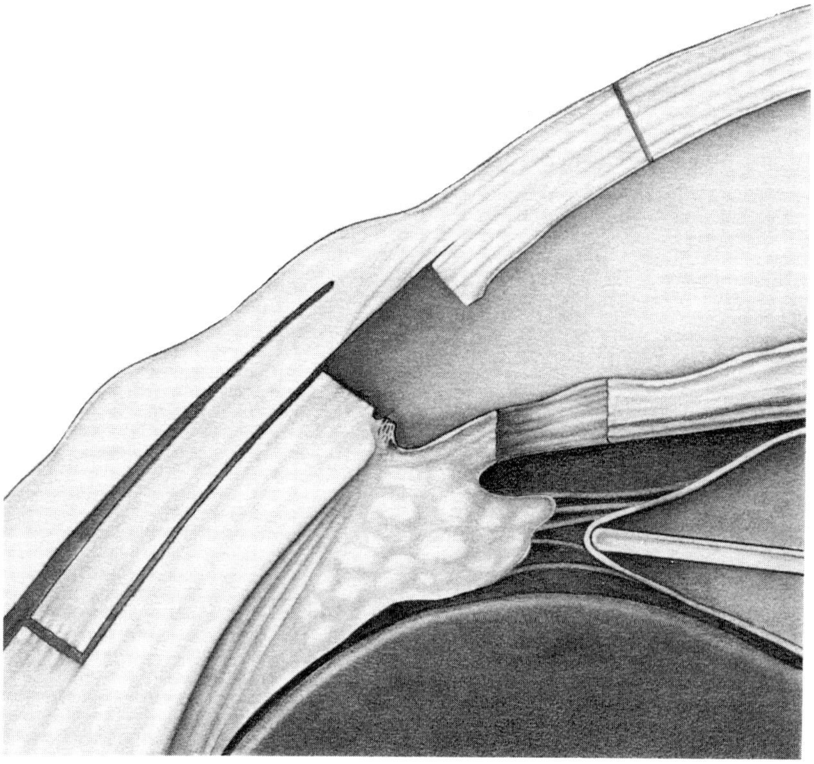

Figure 11–19

12

Cataract Surgery and Intraocular Lens Implantation in an Eye with a Preexisting Filtering Bleb

An approach to cataract surgery in an eye that has a filtration bleb has two goals: (1) to remove the cataract and implant an intraocular lens (IOL) and (2) to preserve the integrity and functioning of the bleb. As a larger number of patients who have had functioning blebs require cataract surgery, the considerations in this chapter will assume greater significance.

Figure 12–1. There are four alternative incision sites for extracapsular cataract surgery in the presence of a filtering bleb. These are (1) anterior to the bleb in clear cornea, (2) temporally, (3) inferiorly, and (4) through the bleb area. I have opted for the incision anterior to the bleb in clear cornea, since it is the orientation that the surgeon is accustomed to and presents only minor alterations in terms of anatomy.

Figure 12–2. If the bleb has been positioned superonasally as the primary procedure, it is most desirable to make the incision superotemporally, using the surgeon's usual technique. This requires only a slight change in the position of the surgeon to perform the procedure.

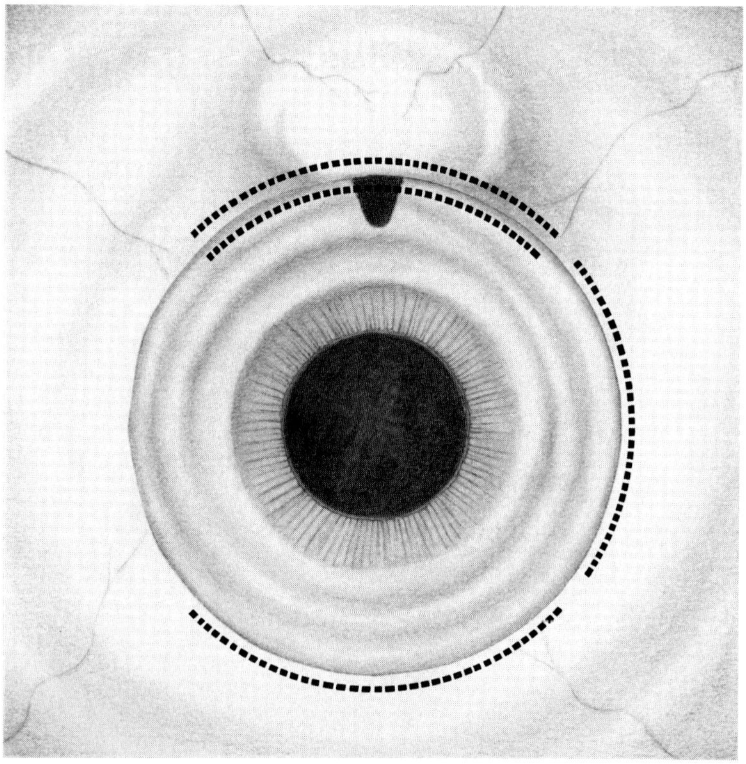

Figure 12–1

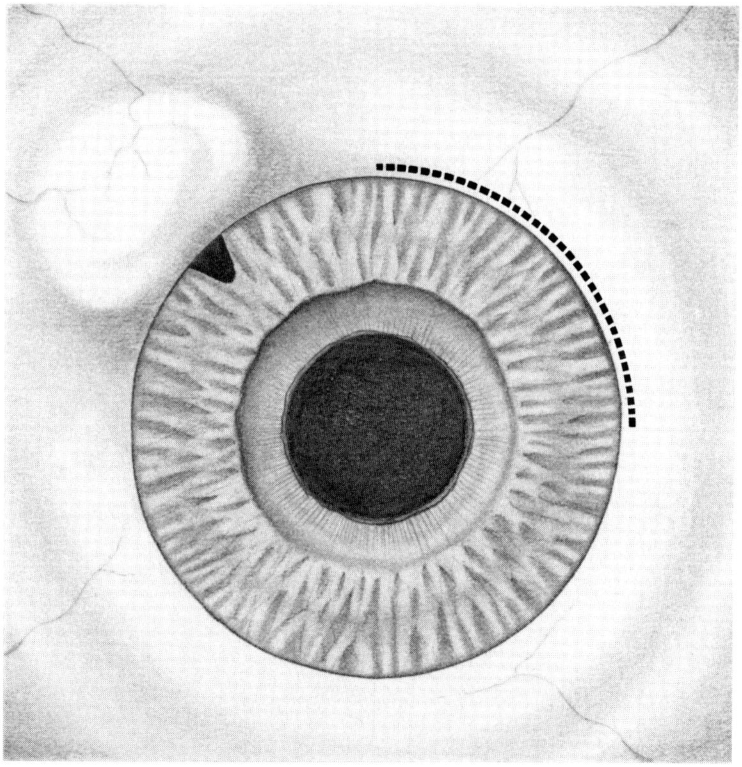

Figure 12–2

Figure 12–3. If the bleb is positioned at 12 o'clock, an incision anterior to the bleb made through the cornea just inside the vascular arcade is chosen. This vertical incision is approximately 4 mm in length and slightly curved to match the contour of the rest of the cataract incision to be created later in the procedure.

Figure 12–4. A viscoelastic agent is introduced into the anterior chamber to deepen it and to protect the endothelium. This material should be introduced slowly and should fill the inferior portion of the chamber initially to displace aqueous from this site.

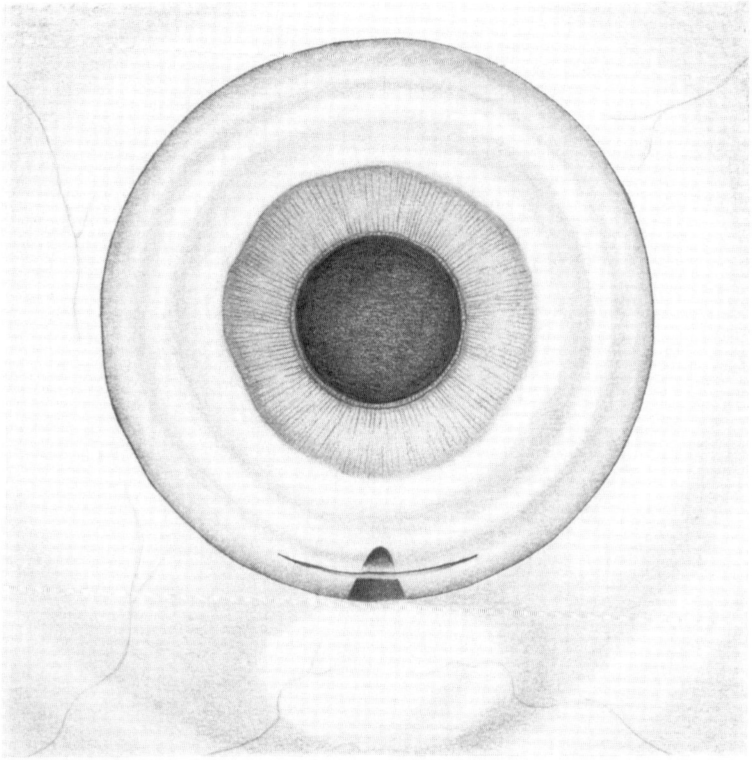

Figure 12–3

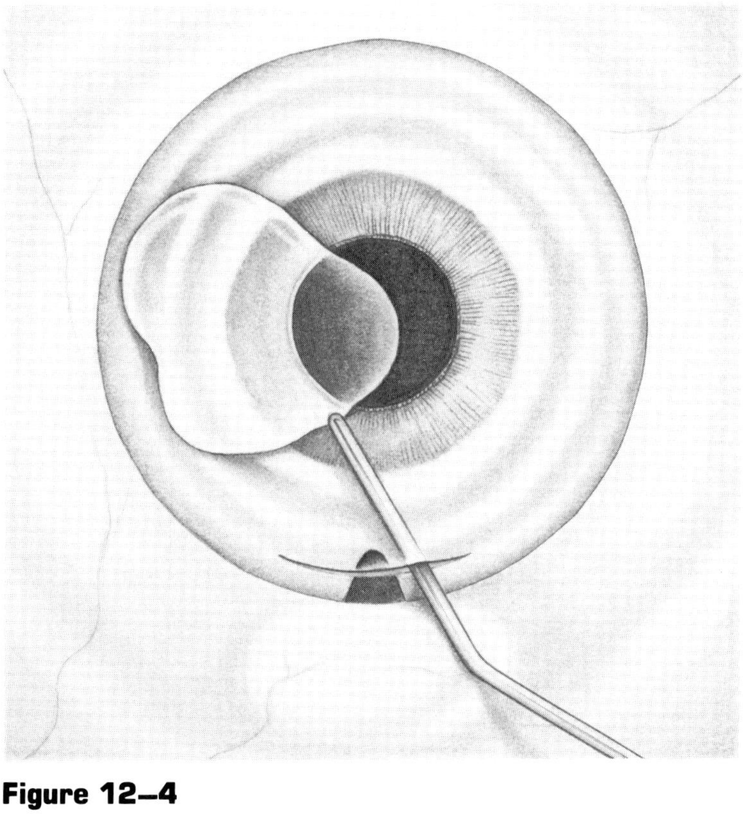

Figure 12–4

Figure 12–5. In many instances, eyes with prior filtering blebs have miotic pupils, either because of posterior synechiae or from chronic miotic therapy. A spatula introduced through the preexisting iridectomy gently breaks the posterior synechiae. A scissors blade is then placed under the iris, and the peripheral iridectomy is converted to a radial sphincterotomy. A small inferior sphincterotomy also is done at this time to ensure adequate access to the inferior portion of the anterior capsule.

Figure 12–6. Additional viscoelastic material is injected into the anterior chamber to widen the pillars of the iris and further deepen the chamber. It is important to have good visualization of the inferior portion of the anterior capsule so that a symmetrical anterior capsulectomy is created. This will prevent late upward decentration of the IOL.

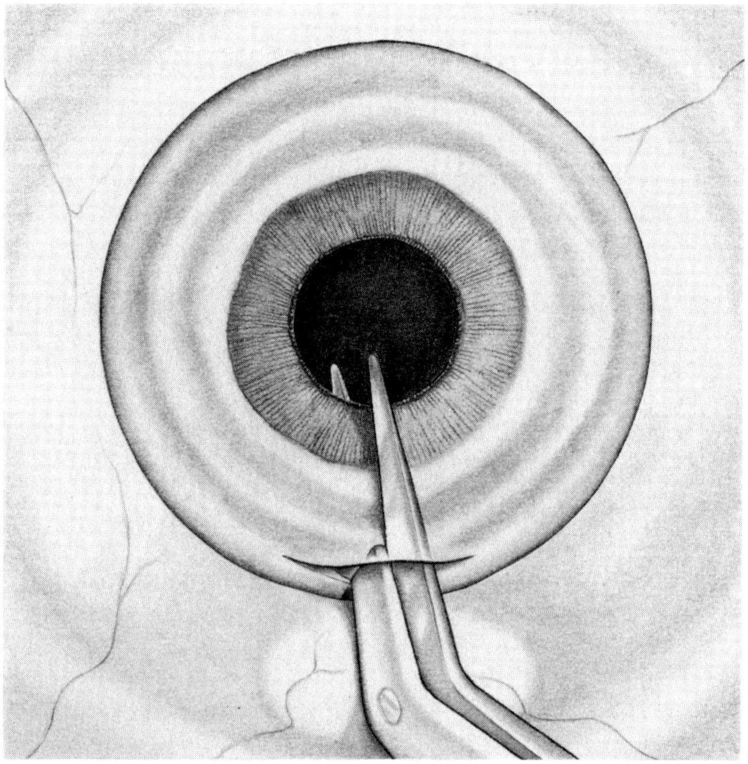

Figure 12–5

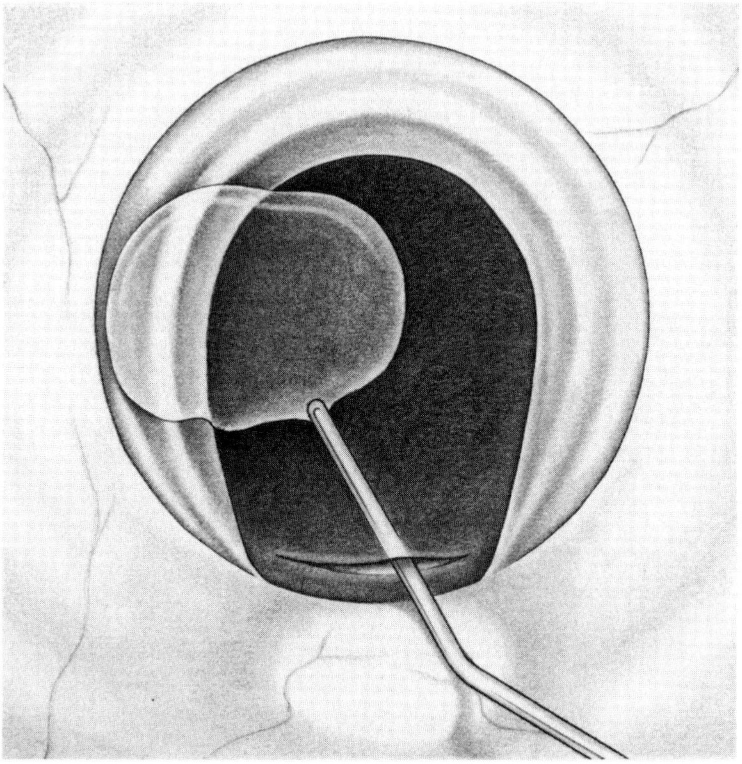

Figure 12–6

Figure 12–7. The anterior capsulectomy of the surgeon's choice is then performed. One can do a standard can-opener technique (**A**), an intercapsular or envelope technique (**B**), or a continuous tear circular capsulectomy, the so-called capsulorrhexis.

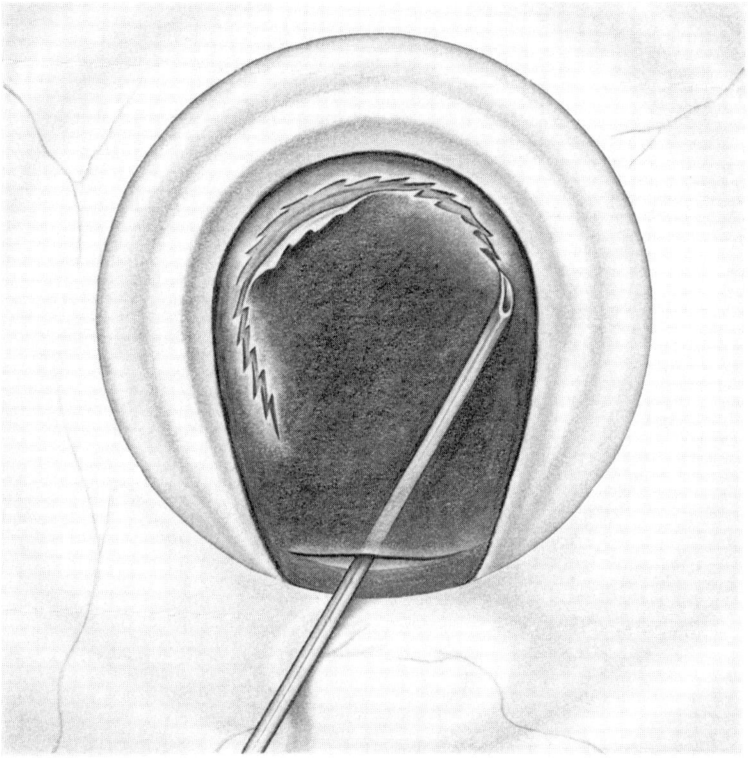

Figure 12–7A

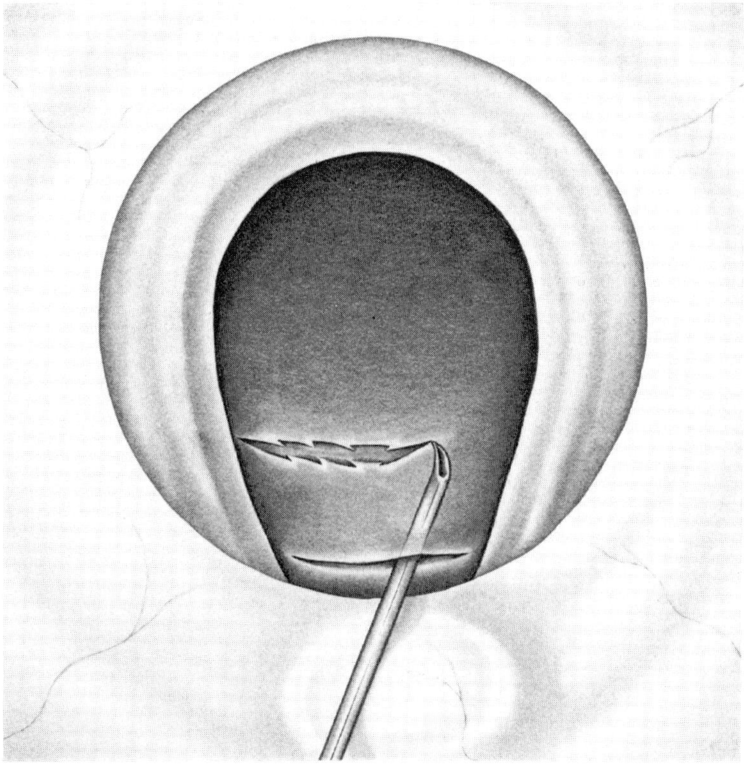

Figure 12–7B

Figure 12–8. The 4-mm incision is enlarged to either side to complete the cataract wound. It is essential to create an adequately sized incision, which may have to be somewhat larger than the standard extracapsular corneoscleral incision. The orientation should be vertical, since a bevelled incision is smaller on its inner aspect than on its outer one.

Figure 12–9. Nucleus removal is performed by the favored technique of the surgeon. Here, nucleus expression is done with gentle pressure applied to the 6 o'clock area just inside the limbus and at 12 o'clock at the wound edge.

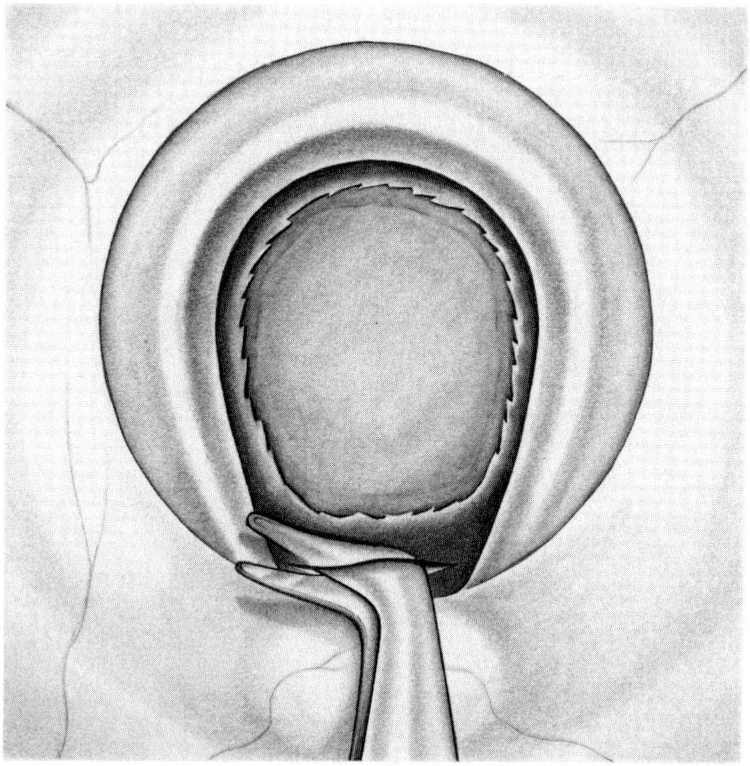

Figure 12–8

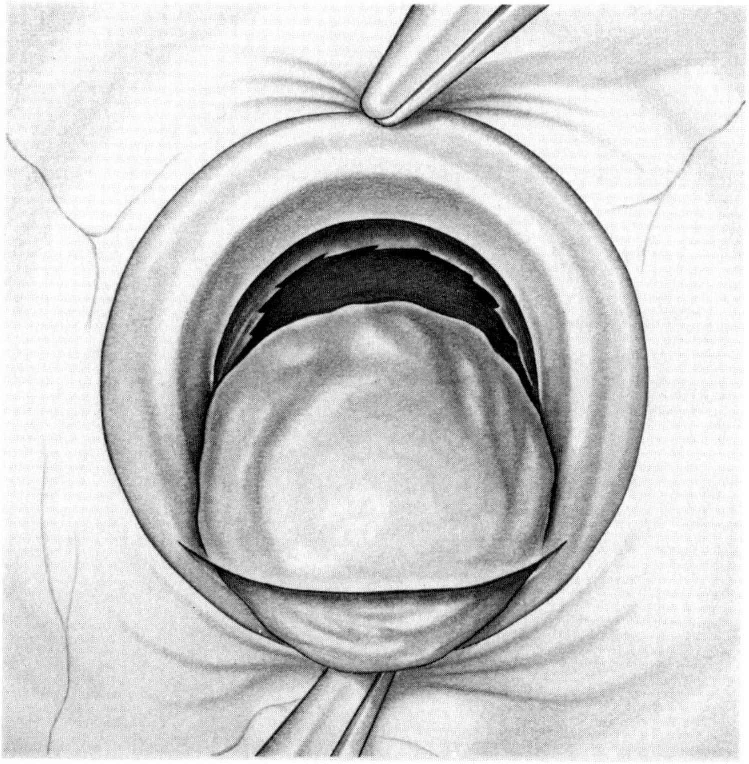

Figure 12–9

Figure 12–10. In preparation for irrigation and aspiration, the peripheral portions of the incision are closed with permanent 10-0 nylon suture, and a temporary suture, to be removed later, is placed at 12 o'clock. Sufficient space is measured between (**A**) and (**B**) to permit smooth introduction of the IOL once the 12 o'clock suture is removed.

Figure 12–11. Irrigation and aspiration of cortical materials are performed by the preferred technique, and the posterior capsule and capsular fornices are polished to remove residual cortex and cells.

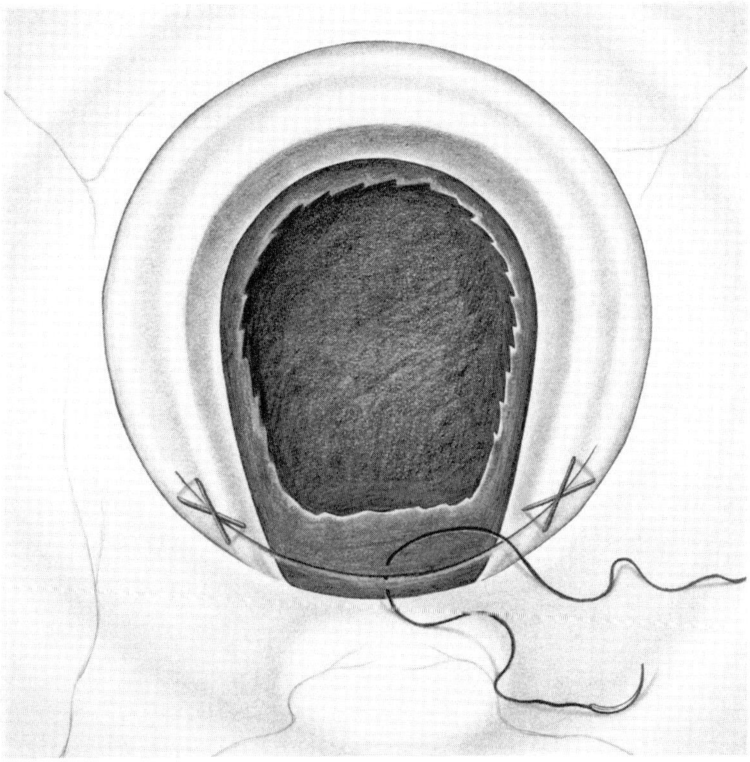

Figure 12–10

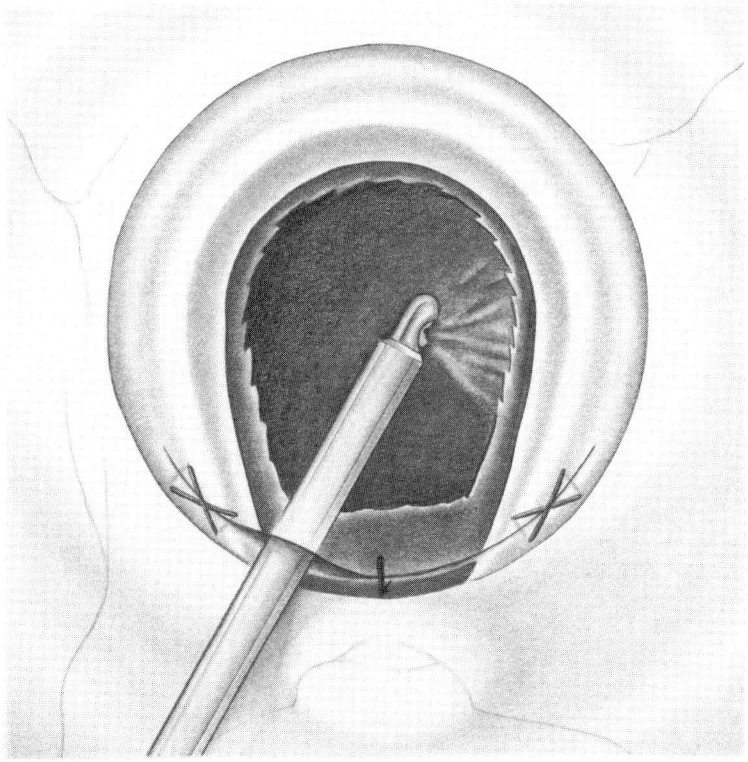

Figure 12–11

Figure 12–12. A. Viscoelastic material is injected to fill the capsular bag. It is desirable to implant the IOL within the bag so that it remains sequestered from the uveal tissue and is distinct from the filtration site. **B.** With the intracapsular (envelope) technique, the superior and inferior flaps of the capsule are still maintained at this point so that, for all intents and purposes, a capsular bag implantation is ensured.

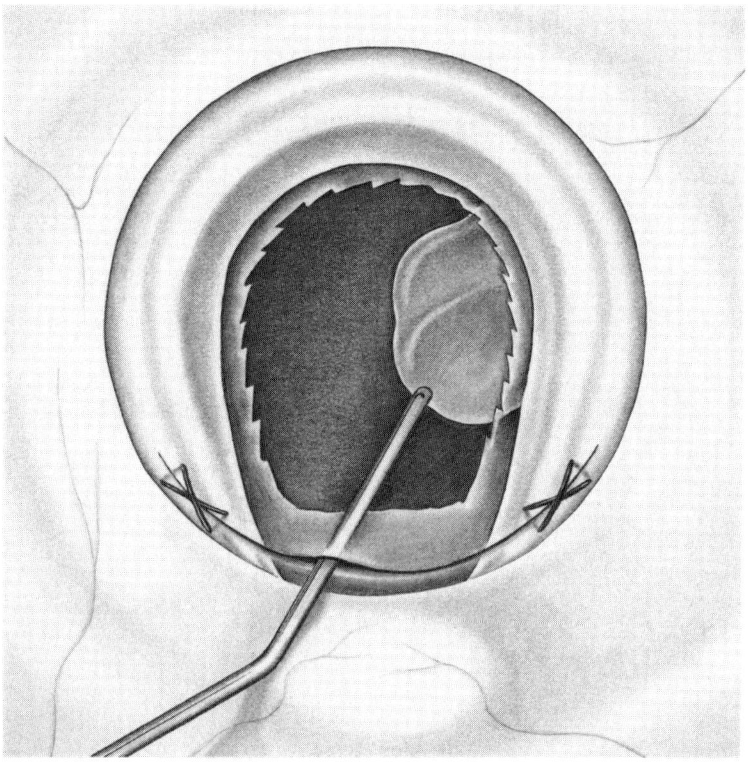

Figure 12–12A

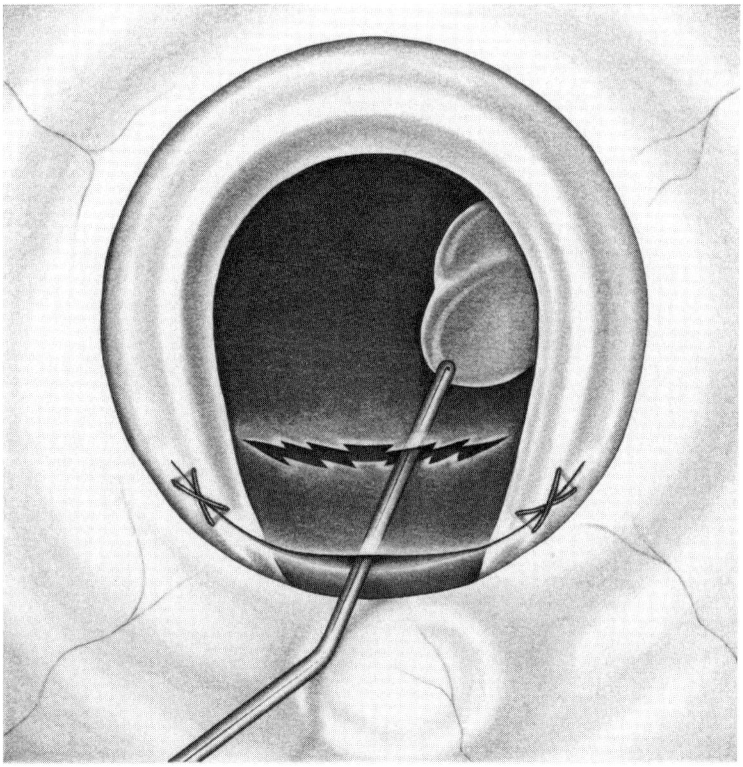

Figure 12–12B

Figure 12–13. The IOL is implanted in three steps. The optic is securely grasped to guide the inferior loop into the inferior capsular fornix. This step is similar for both the can-opener (**A**) and envelope (**B**) capsulotomies.

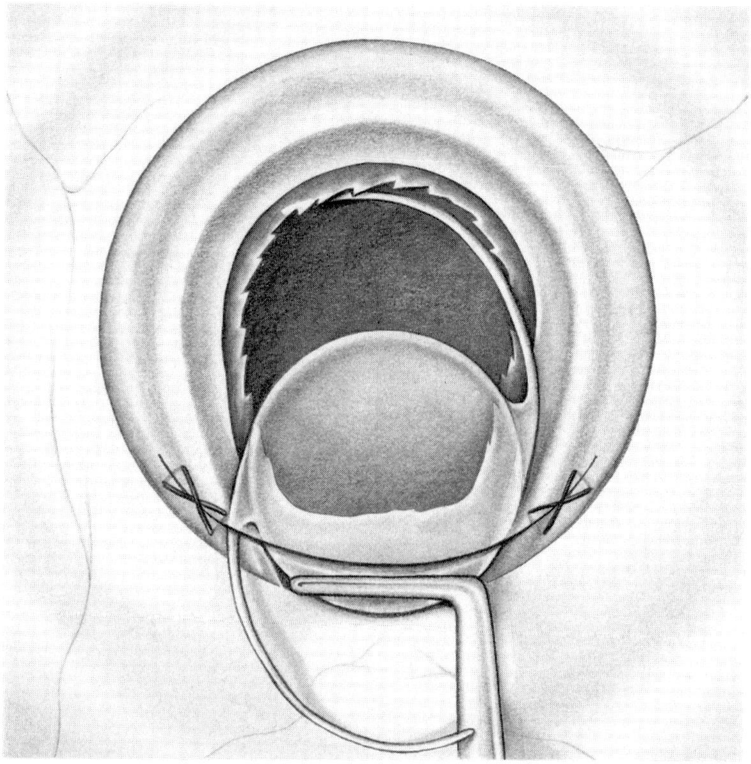

Figure 12–13A

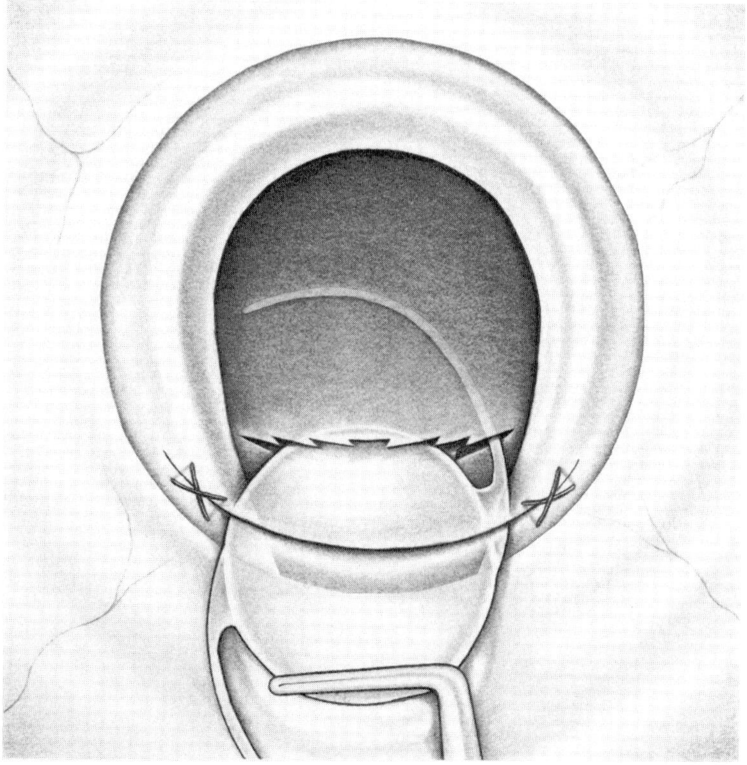

Figure 12–13B

Figure 12–14. The entire optic is placed within the capsular bag, manipulating the lens with the superior haptic. Having the inferior loop and optic within the capsular bag facilitates placing the superior loop.

Figure 12–15. The superior loop of this one-piece PMMA lens implant can be positioned by grasping it with forceps and flexing the loop to place it beneath the superior capsular flap or by rotating the lens with a hook placed at the junction of the loop and the optic, since this 7-mm optic IOL does not have a positioning hole.

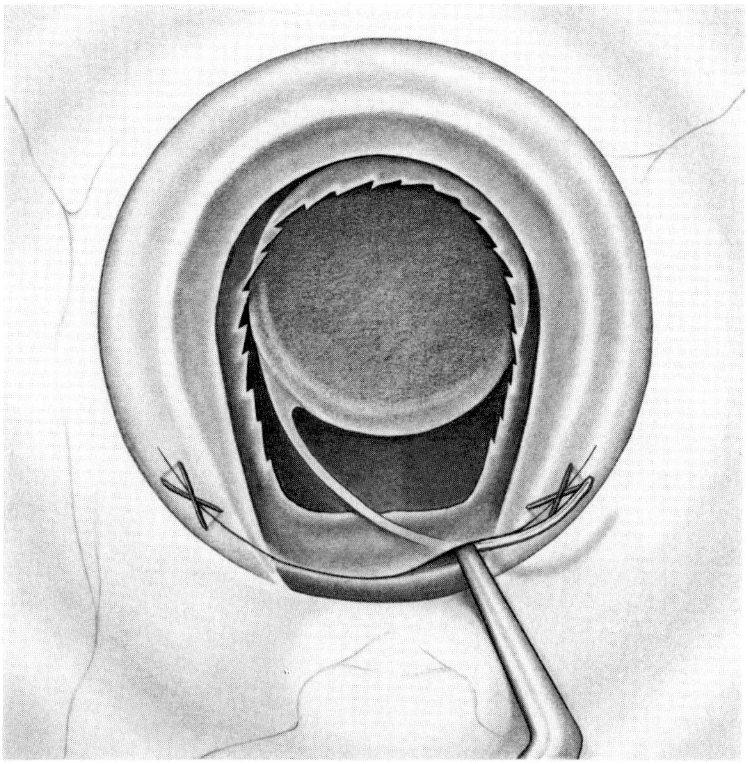

Figure 12–14

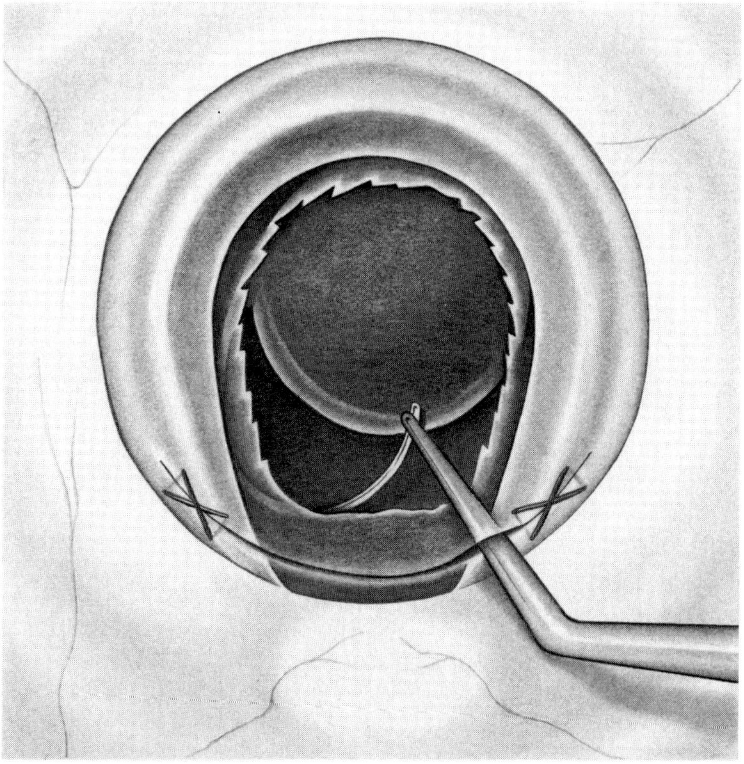

Figure 12–15

Figure 12–16. A. The viscoelastic material is removed with the irrigation–aspiration unit, and the incision is permanently sutured. Generally, the radial iridectomy is not reconstituted and does not result in visual problems. **B.** When the intercapsular or envelope technique has been used, a piece of the anterior capsule is removed before removal of the viscoelastic material by making two incisions in the capsule and a continuous tear inferiorly.

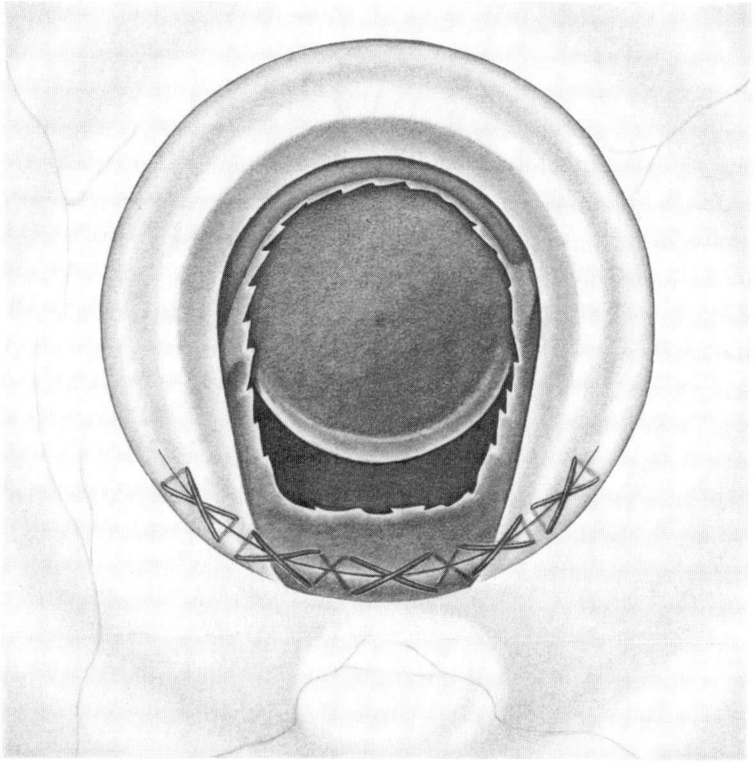

Figure 12–16A

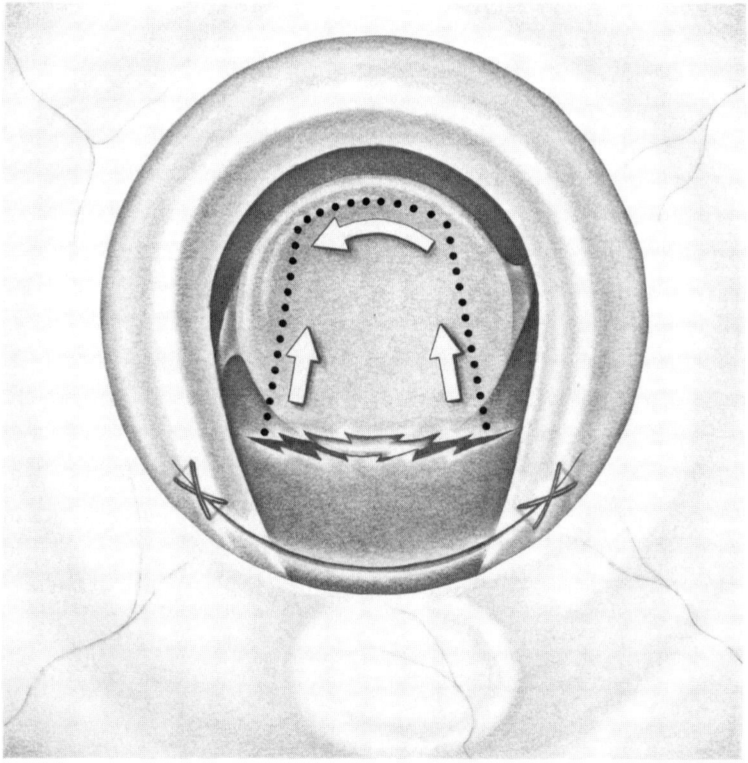

Figure 12–16B

Figure 12–17. In those instances where the surgeon chooses to reconstitute the iris to form a rounded pupil, a 10-0 Prolene suture placed before nucleus removal and looped aside for the remainder of the procedure can now be tied and cut.

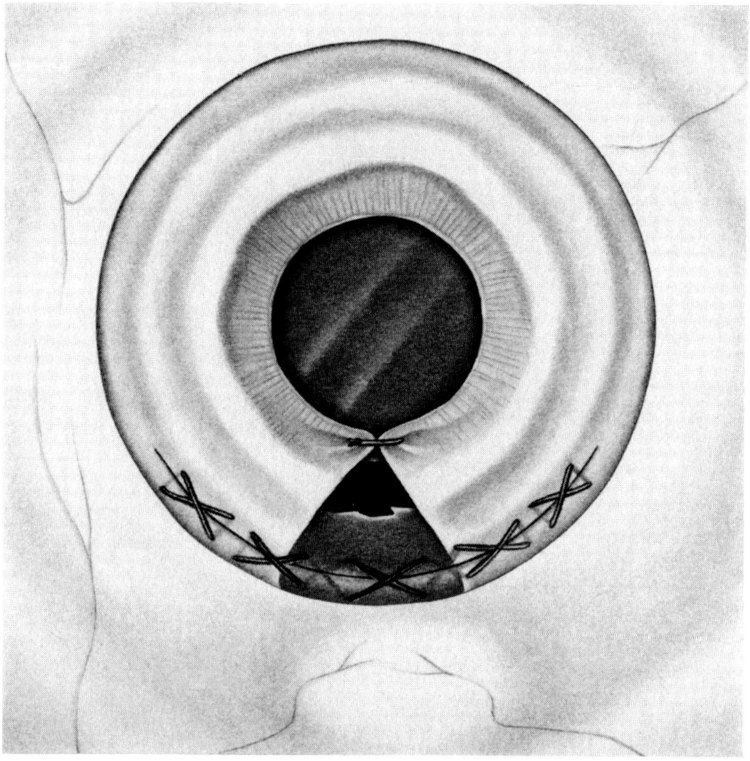

Figure 12–17

13

Repair of the Leaking Bleb

A major complication of filtration procedures is the development of a leaking bleb. Unchecked aqueous loss can produce a shallow to flat anterior chamber, choroidal detachment, and cataract formation. In addition, this complication is of particular concern when a full-thickness procedure has been performed because of the potential for an intraocular infection.

We have found that silk sutures for the conjunctival–corneal portion of the following procedure are advantageous, since they produce a greater inflammatory response to promote a more rapid adhesion of the conjunctiva to corneal tissue and also because they resist retraction of the conjunctival tissue to a greater extent than do nylon sutures.

Figure 13–1. The defect in the bleb is identified by doing a Seidel test. A peritomy incision is made to mobilize the conjunctival tissue at the limbus. Injection of balanced saline solution or, preferably, a viscoelastic material separates the conjunctiva from the underlying tissues. Once a tissue plane has been created, a cannula can be used to lyse any adhesions that may be present. It is desirable to avoid sharp dissection if possible.

Figure 13–2. After the conjunctival tissue is mobilized, a relaxing incision is made through the superior conjunctiva. Tenon's capsule should not be incised at this time. The object is to loosen the conjunctival tissue sufficiently that it can be drawn downward easily. Including Tenon's capsule at this juncture does not add appreciably to achieving this goal. There are some situations, however, where Tenon's capsule must be incised because there is inadequate mobility of the conjunctival tissue.

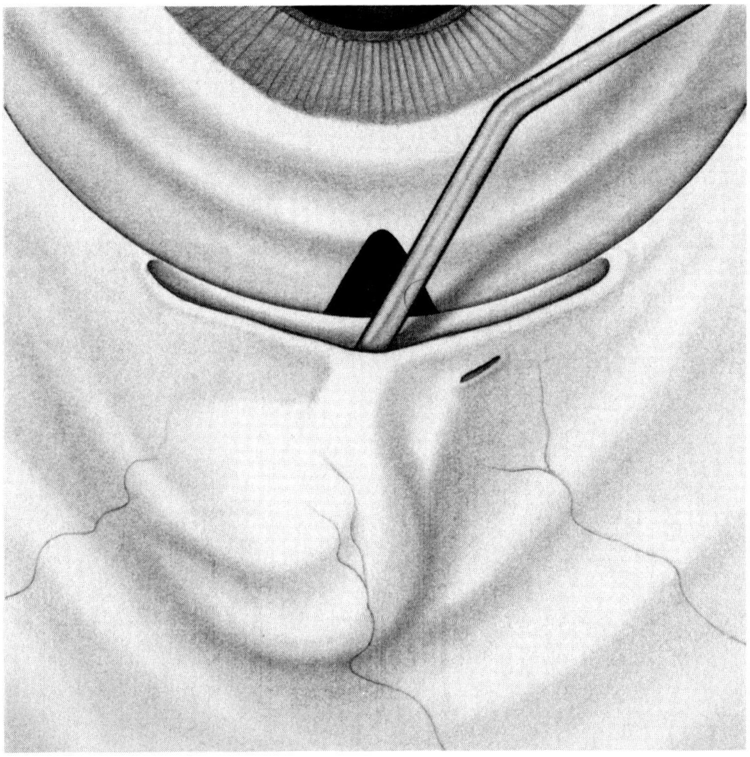

Figure 13–1

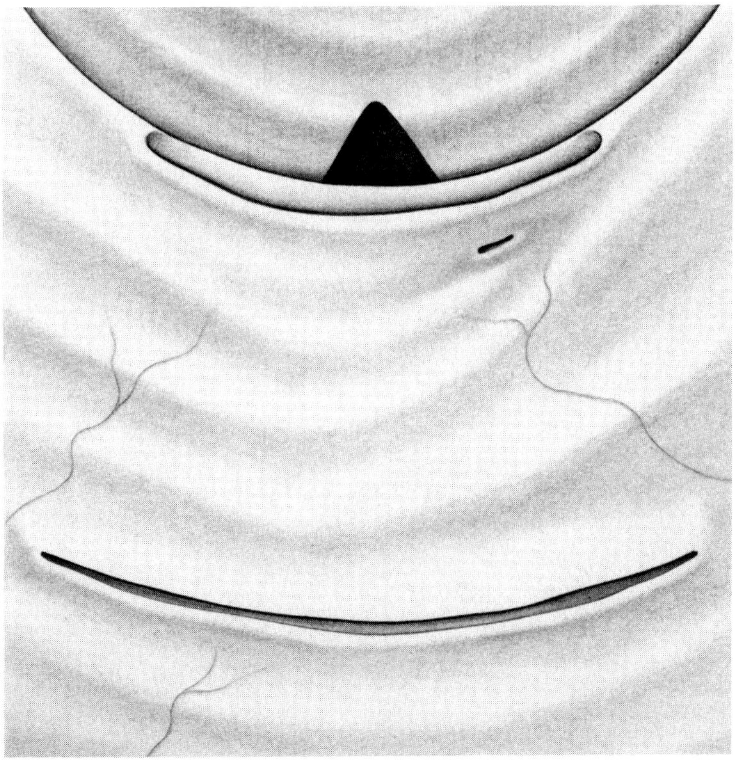

Figure 13–2

Figure 13–3. A vertically oriented, cordlike incision is made in the cornea anterior to the bleb. This incision should be one third to one half of corneal thickness. An incision that is too shallow will not afford the stability required to anchor the conjunctival flap. The incision should be just slightly longer than the extent of the conjunctival incision.

Figure 13–4. Several double-armed 8-0 silk mattress sutures are placed near the edge of the mobilized conjunctival flap and carried through the depth of the corneal incision to merge from the clear cornea. A sufficient number of double-armed sutures are inserted to ensure secure placement of the conjunctival flap. Too few sutures can cause puckering of the conjunctival tissue and an inadequate sealing at the corneal grooved incision.

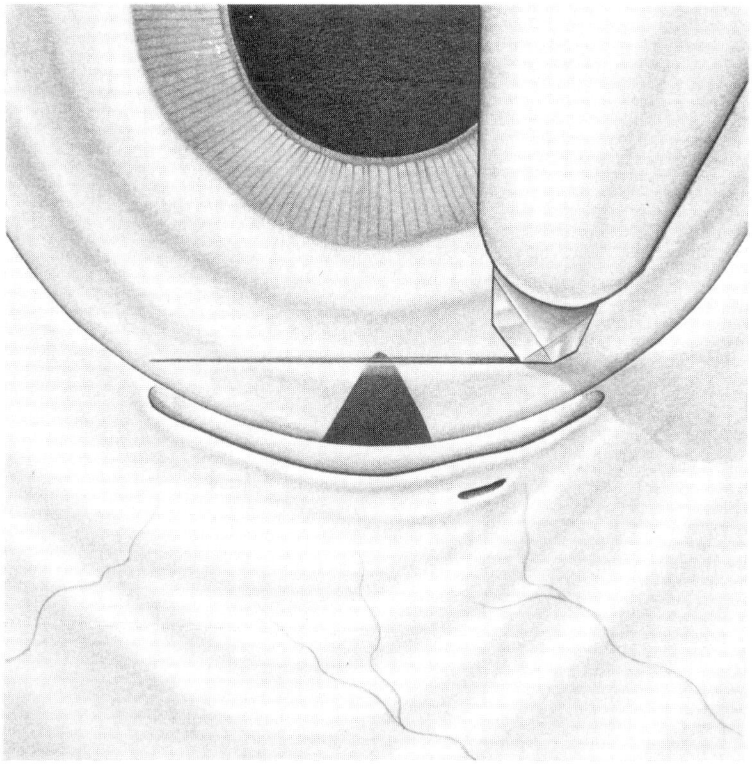

Figure 13–3

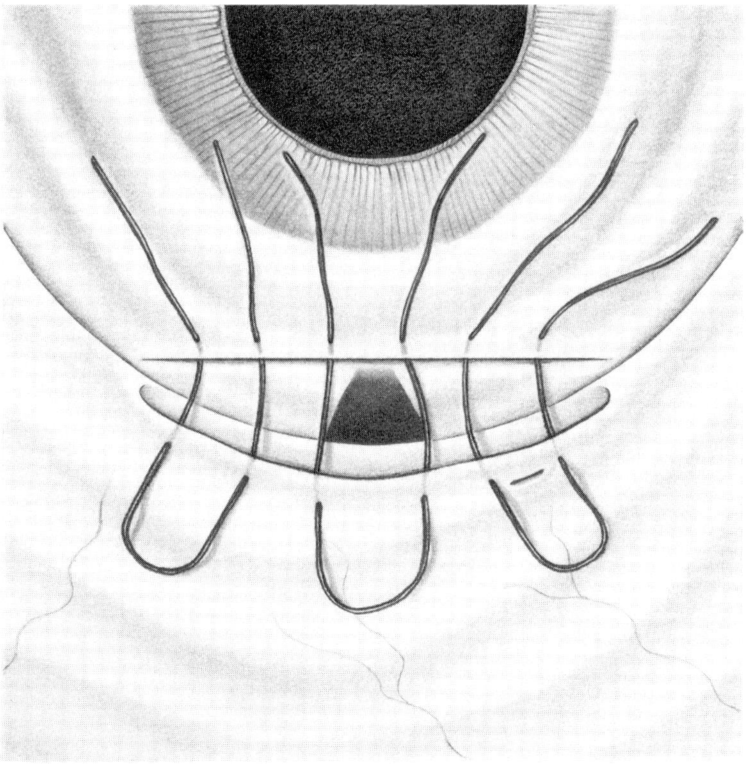

Figure 13–4

Figure 13–5. This cross-sectional view depicts the suture placement through the conjunctival flap and passage of the free end of the suture through the base of the groove. Deep placement of the suture in the corneal tissue is an important factor in anchoring the conjunctival flap in the grooved incision.

Figure 13–6. The anterior tongue of the conjunctival tissue is brought down into the incision, and each of the double-armed sutures is loosely approximated. It is best not to pull on the sutures alone when bringing the conjunctival flap into the grooved incision but to use tissue forceps to pull the conjunctival tissue downward also. The sutures are then tied definitively.

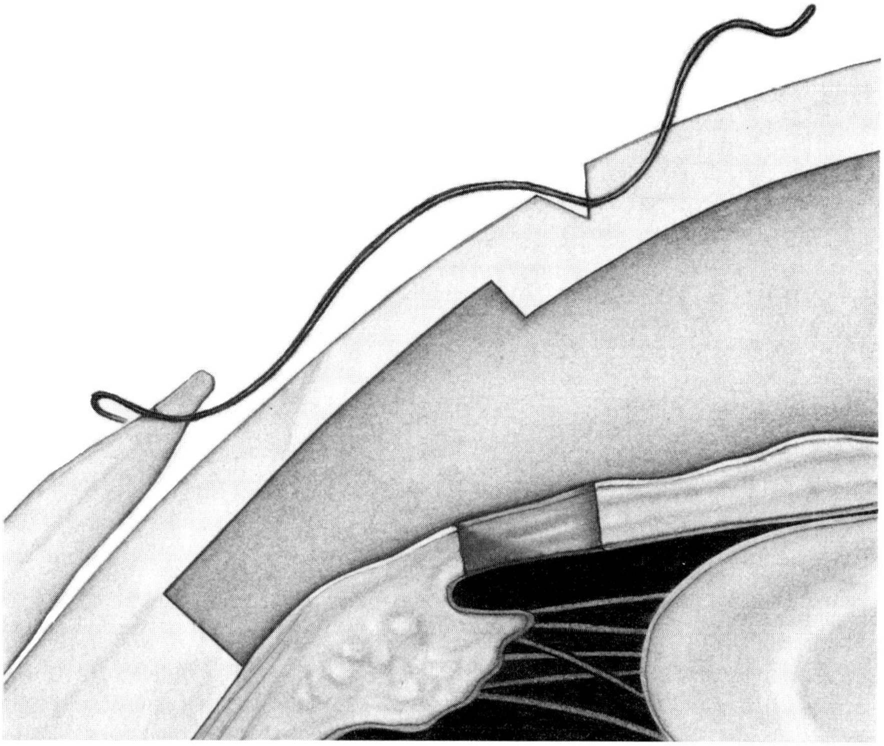

Figure 13–5

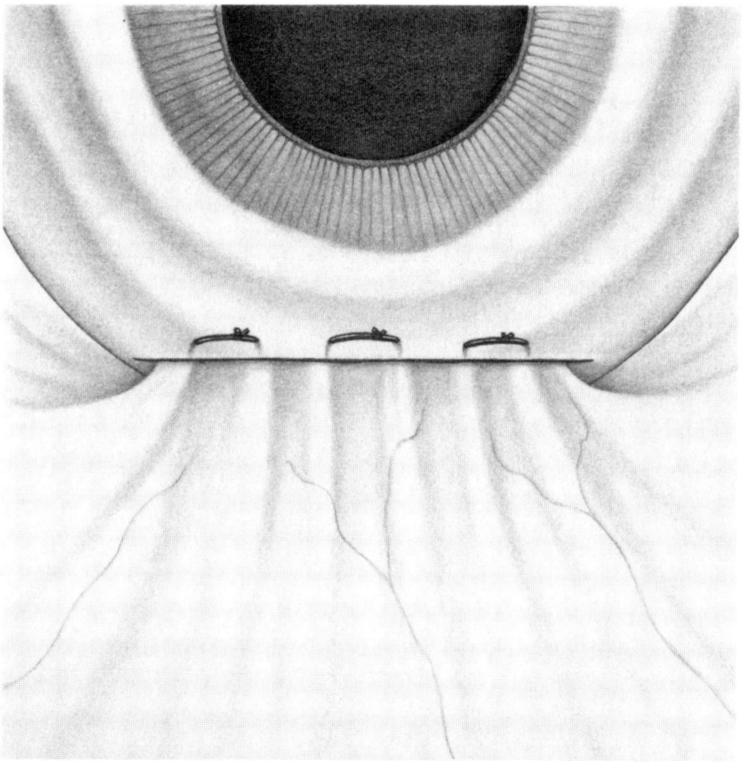

Figure 13–6

Figure 13–7. The conjunctival tissue is closed with a continuous running Vicryl suture. This closure does not have to be tight but should approximate the tissue without producing tension on the conjunctival flap.

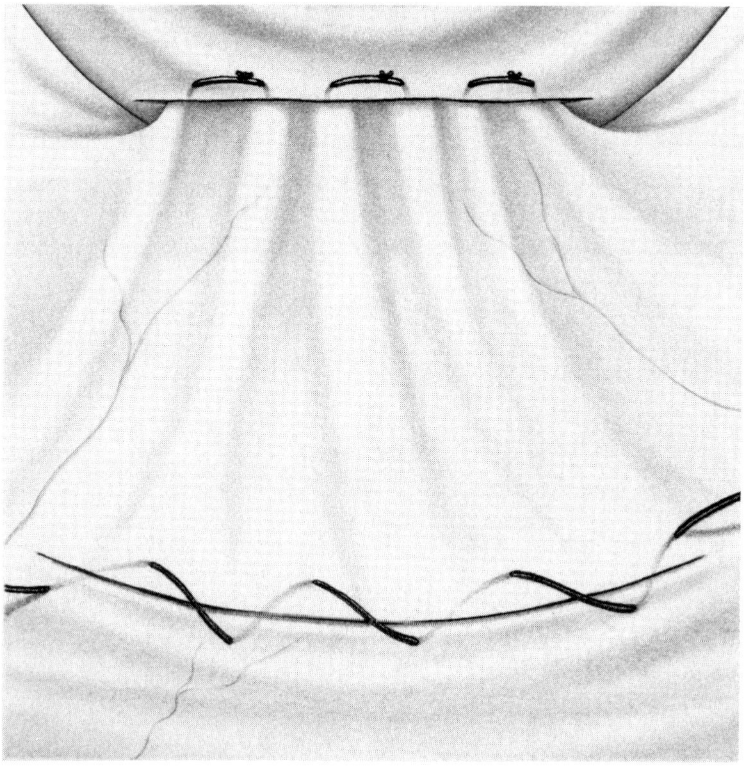

Figure 13–7

14

Glaucoma Filtering Valve Implant to 180 Degree Scleral Explant

Carl B. Camras, Theodore Krupin, and Steven M. Podos

Conventional filtering surgery in certain patients with glaucoma is at high risk for failure. These situations include failure with previous conventional filtering operations, neovascular glaucoma, aphakic glaucomatous eyes without intact posterior capsules, glaucoma in young or black patients, uveitic glaucoma, other secondary glaucomas with extensive peripheral anterior synechiae, and eyes that have undergone previous intraocular or conjunctival surgery. Although most filtering procedures that fail do so on the basis of external scarring at the level of the lamellar scleral flap, Tenon's capsule, or overlying conjunctiva, such operations in neovascular glaucoma also may fail because of growth of fibrovascular tissue over the internal sclerostomy site in the angle.

A long, unidirectional, pressure-sensitive valve attached to a scleral explant provides optimal conditions to maintain filtration in refractory glaucoma cases. The proximal end of the implant is inserted into the anterior chamber through the limbus under a lamellar scleral flap, and its distal end is secured in the groove of an inverted Silastic band placed beneath the rectus muscles extending 180 degrees around the equator of the globe. The proximal end effectively displaces the internal sclerostomy site from the angle structures to a more central position in the anterior chamber, thus avoiding internal occlusion by a fibrovascular membrane. The area for external filtration is diverted far posteriorly, where there seems to be less of a chance for failure from external factors compared with anterior filtration near the limbus. The large area of encapsulation provided by the scleral explant also helps prevent failure from external factors by allowing sufficient aqueous flow across the capsule to reduce IOP.

We use this procedure in neovascular glaucoma usually only after failure with a short glaucoma filtering valve or a Molteno implant and in other glaucomas only after previous failure of at least two standard glaucoma filtering procedures, usually one partial-thickness and one full-thickness procedure. Occasionally, it is used as the primary procedure in neovascular glaucoma.

Supported in part by an unrestricted grant from Research to Prevent Blindness, Inc., New York, NY, as well as NEI grants EY07865, EY01867, and EY05852, National Institutes of Health, Bethesda, MD.

Figure 14–1. A. The Silastic implant has an inner diameter of 0.3 mm and an outer diameter 0.64 mm. The Supramid fixation struts are attached 20 mm from the distal valve end of the device. **B.** The proximal end of the implant is cut with a bevel directed anteriorly so that the open tube extends 1–4 mm into the anterior chamber. **C.** The distal end of the implant has horizontal and vertical slits at right angles, functioning as a unidirectional, pressure-sensitive valve with an opening pressure of 10–12 mm Hg and a closing pressure of 8–10 mm Hg.

Figure 14–2.A. With the groove side of a No. 220 Silastic explant positioned anteriorly, a 16-gauge angiocatheter is inserted through one side from the grooved center in an outward direction. **B.** The central trocar is withdrawn, leaving the plastic angiocatheter in position. The distal valve end of the implant is inserted through the end of the angiocatheter. **C.** The angiocatheter is withdrawn, leaving the implant securely in place through one side of the scleral explant. Before withdrawal of the angiocatheter, the implant is oriented so that the Supramid struts are parallel to the explant for fixation to the sclera.

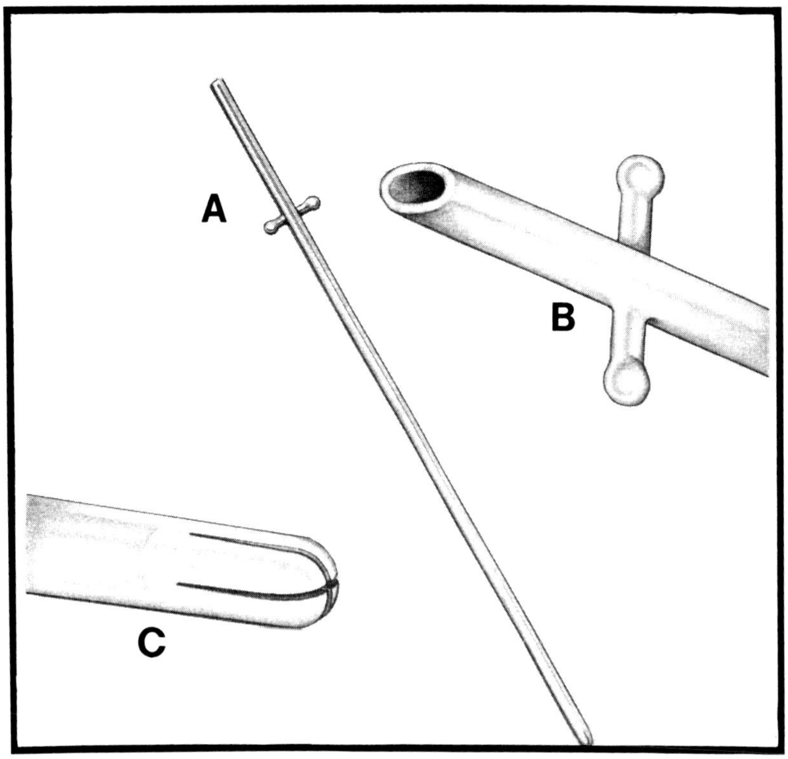

Figure 14–1

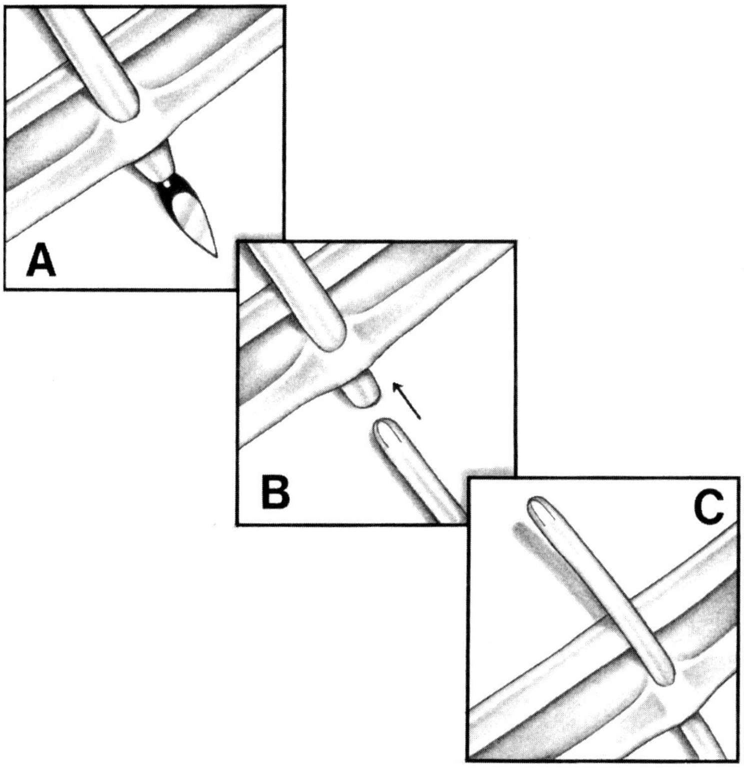

Figure 14–2

Figure 14–3. The implant within the scleral explant is positioned so that the distance between the Supramid fixation struts of the implant and its entry into the scleral explant is 8–10 mm.

Figure 14–4. The distal end of the implant is positioned within the groove of the Silastic scleral explant so that there is a gradual bend to one side, preventing kinking and occlusion. The valve end is positioned in the center of the groove and secured in place with two or three interrupted 9-0 or 10-0 nylon or polypropylene sutures passed in a mattress fashion, full-thickness through the explant. The distal fixation suture is placed no closer than 2 mm from the end of the implant to completely avoid the valve.

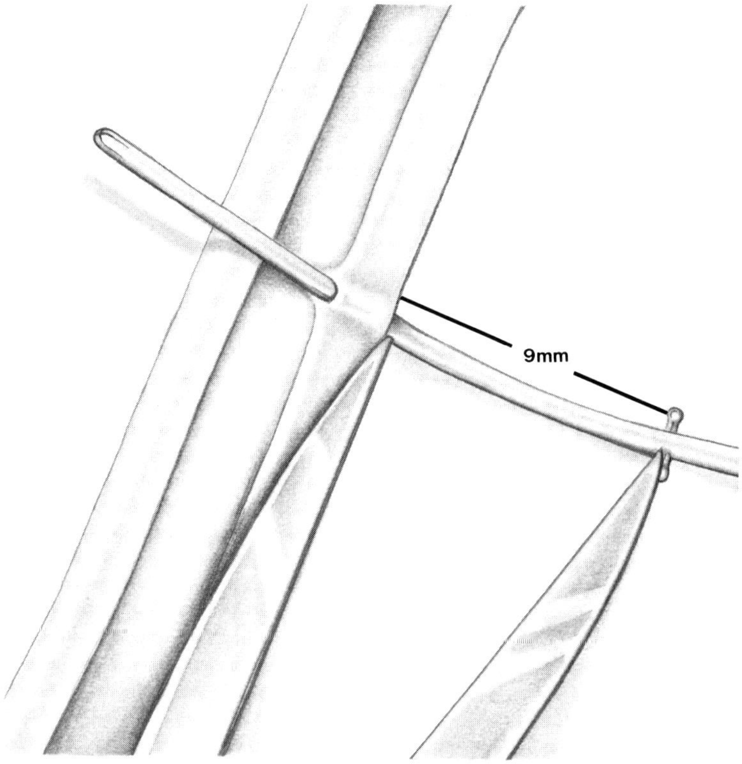

Figure 14–3

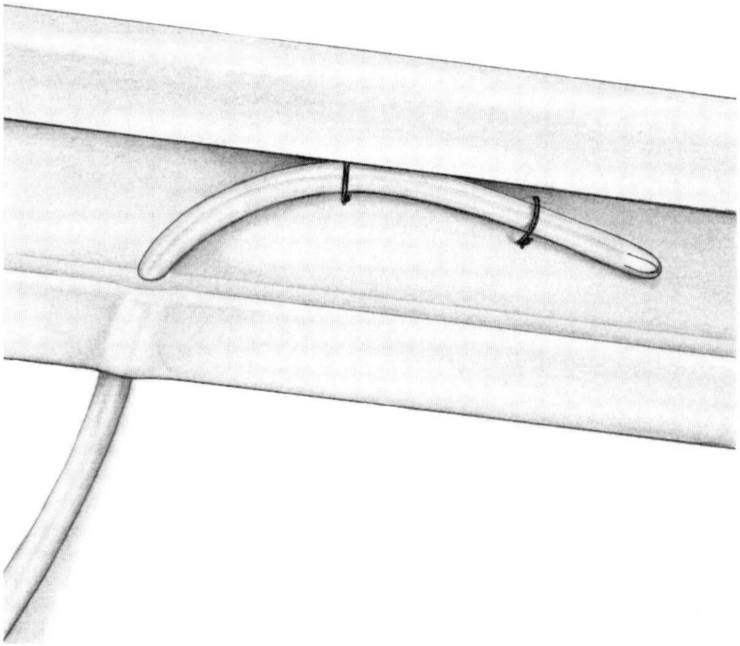

Figure 14–4

Figure 14–5. A 180-degree limbal peritomy is performed, with radial relaxation incisions through the conjunctiva at the end of the peritomy. The conjunctiva is reflected posteriorly, and three rectus muscles are isolated with 2-0 silk sutures. Two 4-0 or 5-0 mersilene mattress sutures are placed in each of the two quadrants between the adjacent rectus muscles. The anterior bites of the mattress sutures are placed 8–10 mm from the limbus, with the second bite 7.5 mm farther posteriorly. The scleral explant is placed beneath the mattress sutures and rectus muscles, with the grooved side toward the sclera. It is centered beneath one rectus muscle and extends to adjacent muscles on each side, with the ends cut with an anterior bevel. It is positioned and secured in place by the mattress sutures so that the implant is centered in a quadrant between adjacent rectus muscles. A 5 × 5 mm lamellar scleral flap, 70%–90% in thickness, is dissected so that the implant is centered under the lamellar scleral flap.

Figure 14–6. After a clear corneal paracentesis track is made in a convenient position away from the lamellar scleral flap, the anterior chamber is filled with sodium hyaluronate. A 20-gauge MVR blade is used to enter the anterior chamber at the limbus, centered beneath the lamellar scleral flap, with the entry parallel to the iris plane.

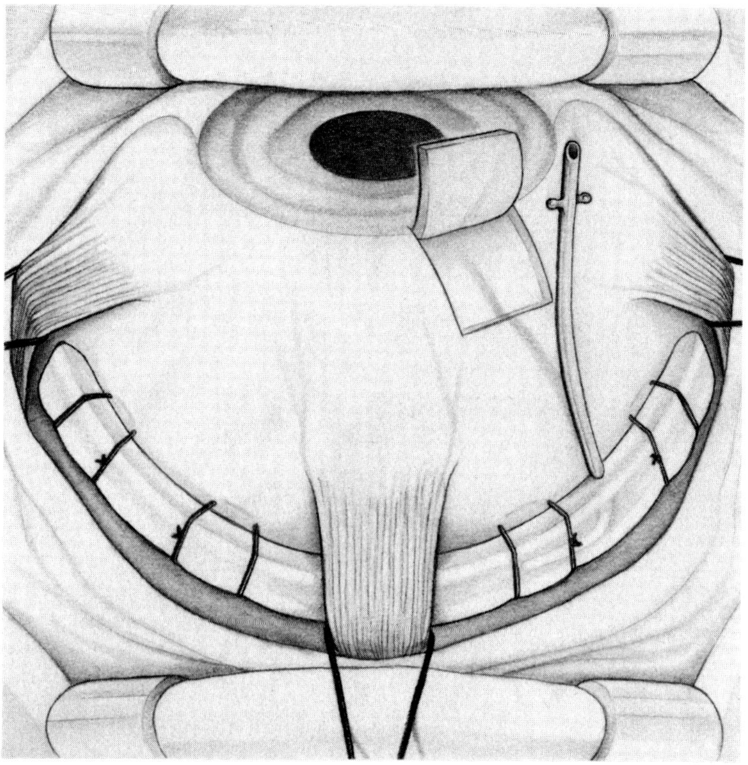

Figure 14–5

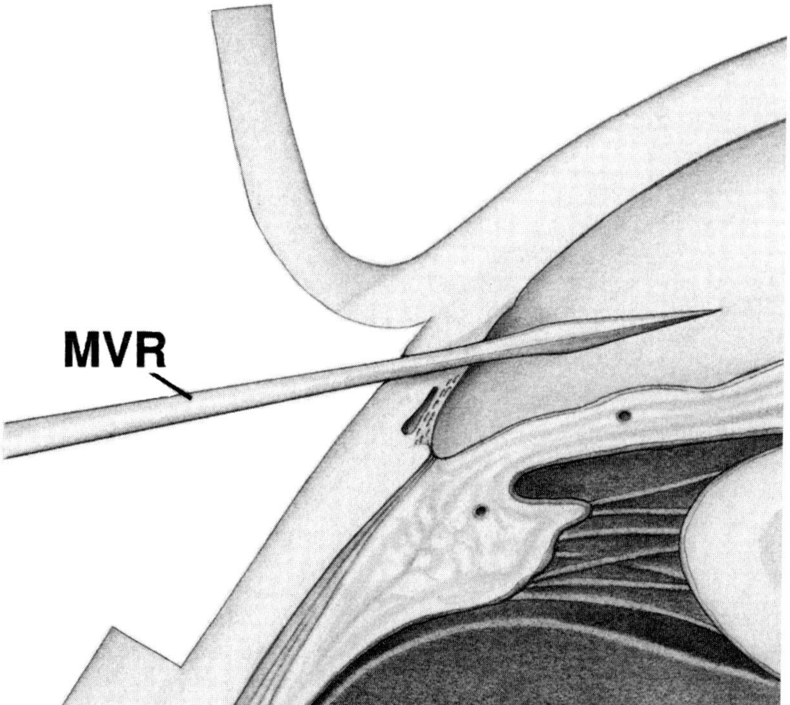

Figure 14–6

Figure 14–7. The proximal end of the implant is cut with an anterior bevel. It is inserted 1–4 mm into the anterior chamber.

Figure 14–8. A double-armed 9-0 or 10-0 nylon suture is passed in a mattress fashion through clear cornea, exiting in the bed of a lamellar scleral flap, with the exit site of the suture determining the posterior position of the fixation struts.

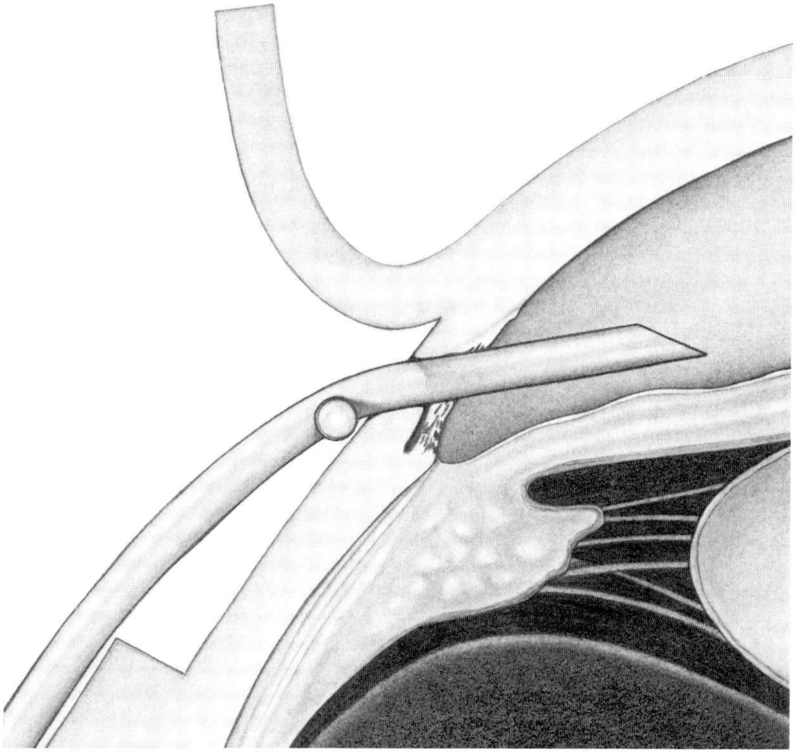

Figure 14–7

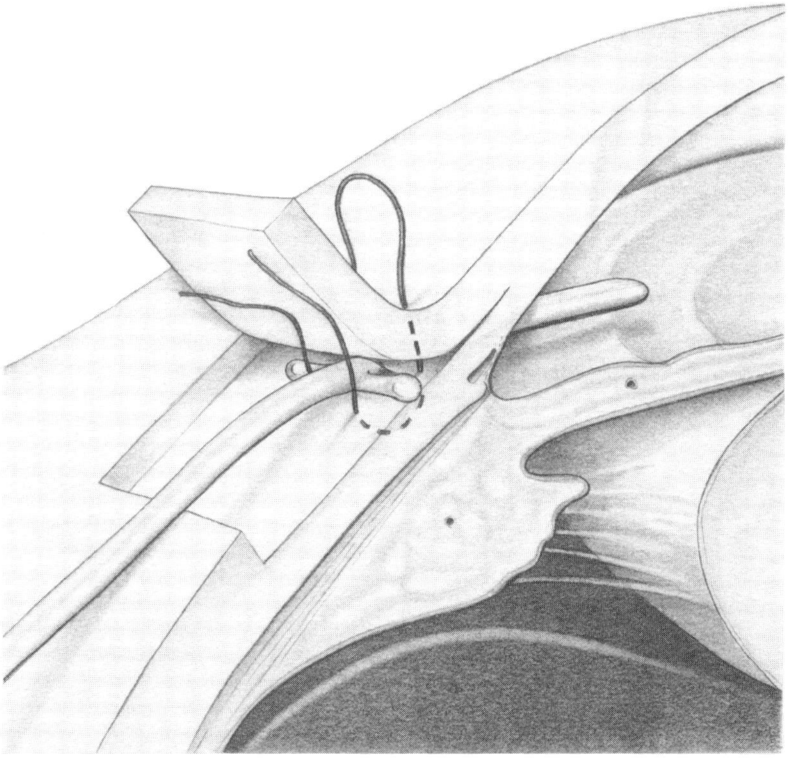

Figure 14–8

Figure 14–9. The nylon mattress suture at the limbus is tied over the implant posterior to the fixation struts, securing it in position. Three to four additional 10-0 nylon sutures are placed to further secure the implant.

Figure 14–10. The lamellar scleral flap is sutured in position over the implant with additional 10-0 nylon sutures, with the posterior corners adequately recessed to prevent excessive pressure of the lamellar scleral flap on the implant, which may lead to erosion. The conjunctiva is reapproximated to the limbus and closed with 8-0 polyglactin sutures.

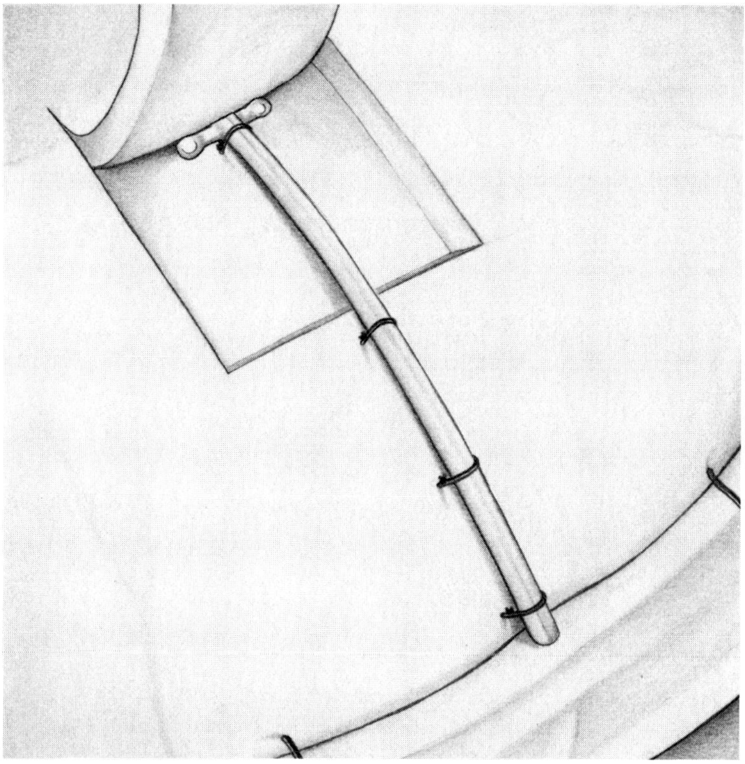

Figure 14–9

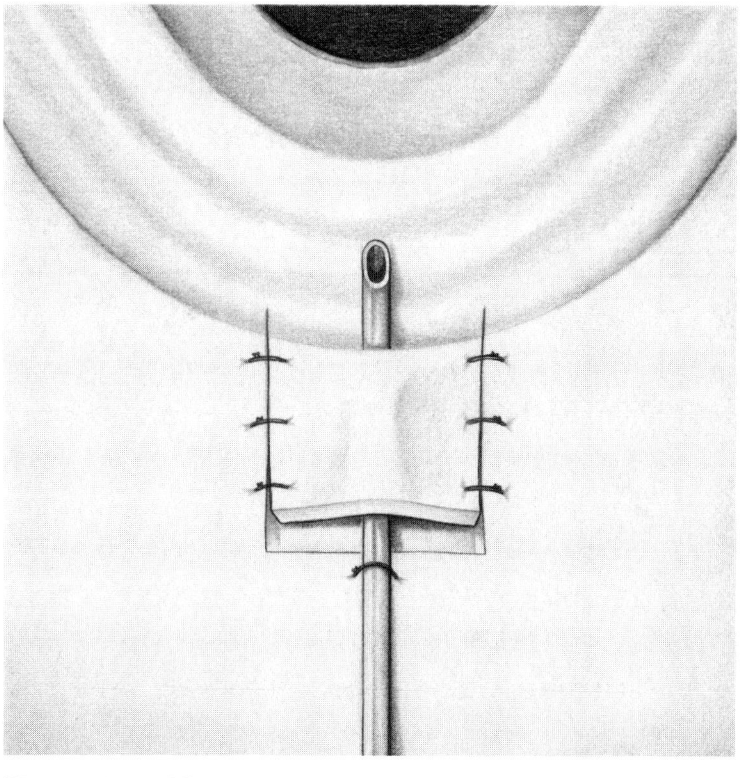

Figure 14–10

15

Glaucoma Surgery and Corneal Transplantation

Kenneth R. Barasch

Medically uncontrolled glaucoma is a complicating factor in many eyes requiring corneal transplantation. Eyes with surgical corneal disease and glaucoma have had cataract extractions, primary or secondary IOL implantation, IOL exchanges, repositioning or removal of an IOL, vitrectomy, glaucoma surgery, and corneal transplants that have already failed. The anterior segment anatomy usually is distorted. Scarred conjunctiva, vitreous in the anterior chamber, malpositioned IOLs, sector and peripheral iridectomy, and peripheral anterior synechiae all affect the choice of surgical approach. All of these factors also may exist in eyes with clear corneal grafts and medically uncontrolled glaucoma that requires surgical management.

Ideally, IOP should be normal or controlled in eyes facing corneal transplantation. Pretransplant glaucoma surgery may be necessary to normalize the IOP. The corneal edema or scar that necessitates the graft usually prevents laser treatment to the iris or filtration angle. The distorted anterior segment anatomy may dictate a less-than-ideal location for a filtration procedure or even preclude it. A small area of open angle with overlying scarred conjunctiva may point the way toward the old and unpredictable cyclodialysis. Cyclodestructive procedures can be done when the distorted anterior segment eliminates all other options. The use of setons, although enticing, is still considered a last resort. When a pretransplant filtration procedure is performed and is successful, the subsequent corneal transplant may lead to its demise. The same holds for cyclodialysis. When cyclodestructive procedures are used, the inflammation produced must subside completely before proceeding with a corneal transplant. This period varies from weeks to many months. Simultaneous corneal transplantation and trabeculectomy can be done in eyes with reasonably good filtration sites. By combining the two procedures, the recovery period is shortened as compared to a two-stage approach, and an encroaching filtration bleb is not a factor when suturing the graft in place.

Posttransplantation medically uncontrollable glaucoma presents the same set of decision-making problems that exists pretransplantation, with the additional and important factor of protecting the clear corneal transplant. The surgical approach producing the least inflammation is preferred to protect the graft endothelium. Ideally, shallowing of the anterior chamber following filtration is to be avoided, particularly in the presence of an anterior chamber IOL. Tighter-than-usual suturing of the trabeculectomy flap minimizes the chance of a shallow chamber. However, it also may decrease the chance of a successful filtration procedure. Later laser release of a tight suture may improve on inadequate filtration secondary to a tight flap (see Fig. 6–29, Hoskins lens). The unpredictable cyclodialysis does not shallow the anterior chamber but may be followed by prolonged hyphema. Late cleft closure of a previously successful cyclodialysis, unfortunately, mimics an attack of angle-closure glaucoma, which can be devastating to the graft endothelium. Laser therapy to the angle through a clear corneal transplant neither shallows the chamber nor produces significant inflammation and can be used if enough unencumbered angle is visible with a gonioprism. It may be inapplicable, however, because of impenetrable anterior synechiae. An inflammation-producing cyclodestructive procedure may be the only alternative. The least cyclodestruction compatible with lowering IOP is our goal. However, to determine this amount currently is impossible, and, therefore, the best approach is to perform the procedure in stages,

The imaginative and seductive glaucoma treatment that has been struggled with for many years involves the use of a valve, which allows aqueous humor to escape from the anterior chamber and to be absorbed in a protected subconjunctival or sub-Tenon's space. This may be the final alternative. Many imaginative designs incorporating pressure-responsive valves have been tried. It is important to remember that these techniques exist. The use of a valve implant is described in Chapter 14.

Figure 15–1. The combined corneal transplantation–IOL exchange–anterior vitrectomy–filtration procedure. The eye is anesthetized by a retrobulbar block, using a mixture of rapid-onset and short-acting local anesthestic and a slower-onset but longer-acting local anesthetic. Intravenous mannitol (2.5–100 mg/kg body weight) is given one half-hour before surgery. A grooved incision to outline the recipient defect is made with the corneal trephine while the globe is still firm so that, once the filtration portion of the procedure has been done, it will be possible to proceed with the corneal transplantation despite the soft eye. In younger patients with more elastic sclera, an eccentrically placed scleral ring to permit an adequate area for filtration is affixed to the globe. Older patients typically have more rigid sclera, so the scleral ring, although beneficial, is not as necessary.

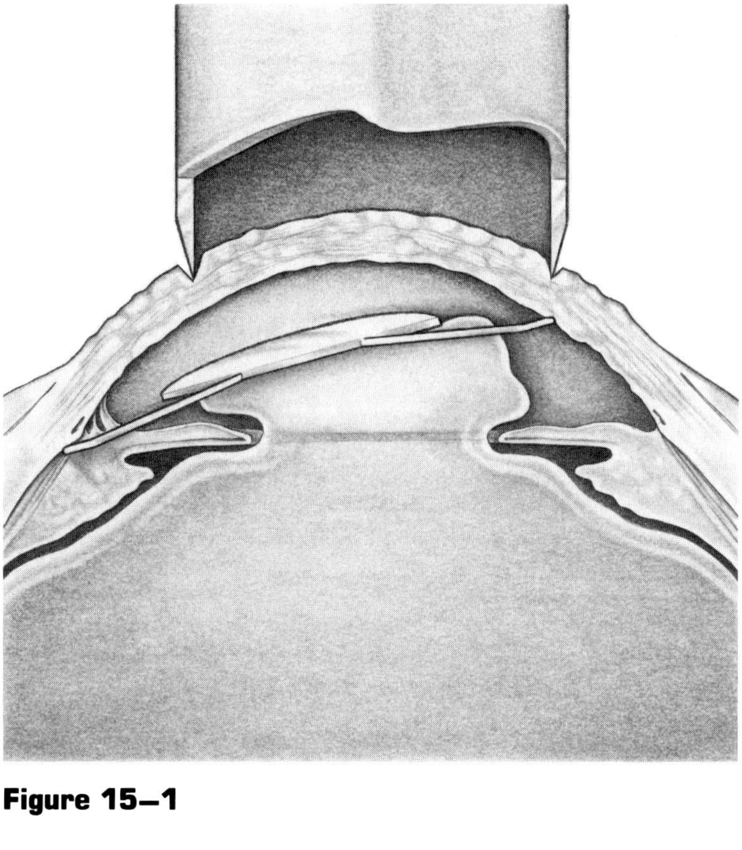

Figure 15–1

Figure 15–2. The major steps of trabeculectomy have been performed. A fornix-based flap has been created, and the superficial scleral flap and deep sclerotomies have been dissected. This three-quarter view of the globe shows the opening into the anterior chamber beneath the deep scleral flap and peripheral iridectomy that already has been performed. The previously created groove outlines the corneal transplant.

Figure 15–3. The recipient corneal button has been removed by first entering the anterior chamber by sharp dissection, then using curved corneal scissors. The anterior chamber IOL to be removed is being grasped with smooth forceps. The inferior haptic is cut free. Since the haptics frequently are enclosed by synechiae, traction on them will cause bleeding. In this case, the superior haptic was free, whereas the inferior haptic was held in place by synechiae. It is important to try to assess the position of the IOL preoperatively in order to formulate a plan for IOL removal. The completed trabeculectomy is seen at lower right.

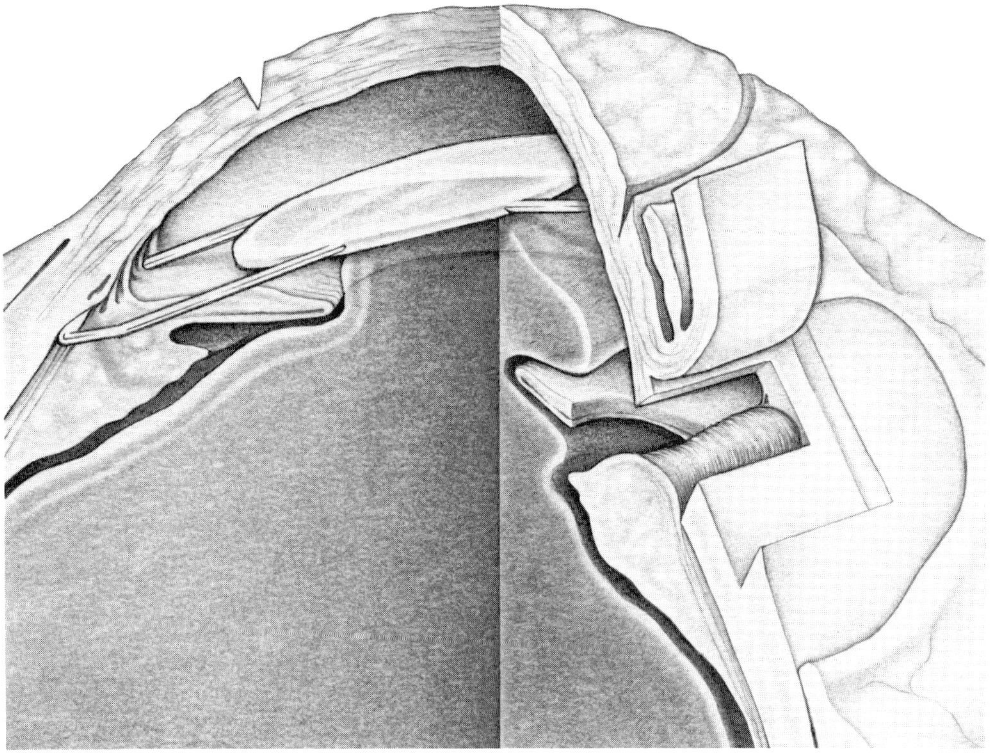

Figure 15–2

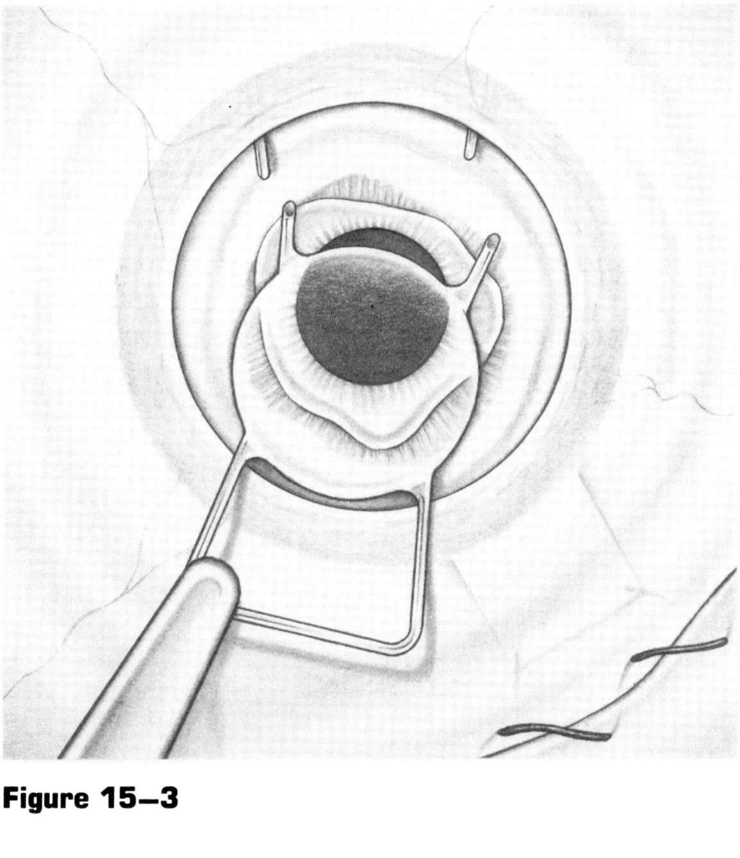

Figure 15–3

Figure 15–4. The inferior haptic is removed by sliding and rotating it from its tunnel of anterior synechiae. Although the haptic is trapped in a cocoon of synechiae, it is not attached to the angle structures or the overlying iris.

Figure 15–5. After removal of the anterior chamber IOL, vitreous may remain in the anterior chamber or herniate through the pupil. The vitrectomy unit is used in the cutting and aspirating mode to remove vitreous from the anterior chamber. Irrigation hydrates the vitreous and often necessitates a more extensive vitrectomy. The use of the scleral ring in younger eyes prevents scleral collapse and vitreous presentation. When vitreous is present in the anterior chamber, a vitrectomy to clear this structure is performed.

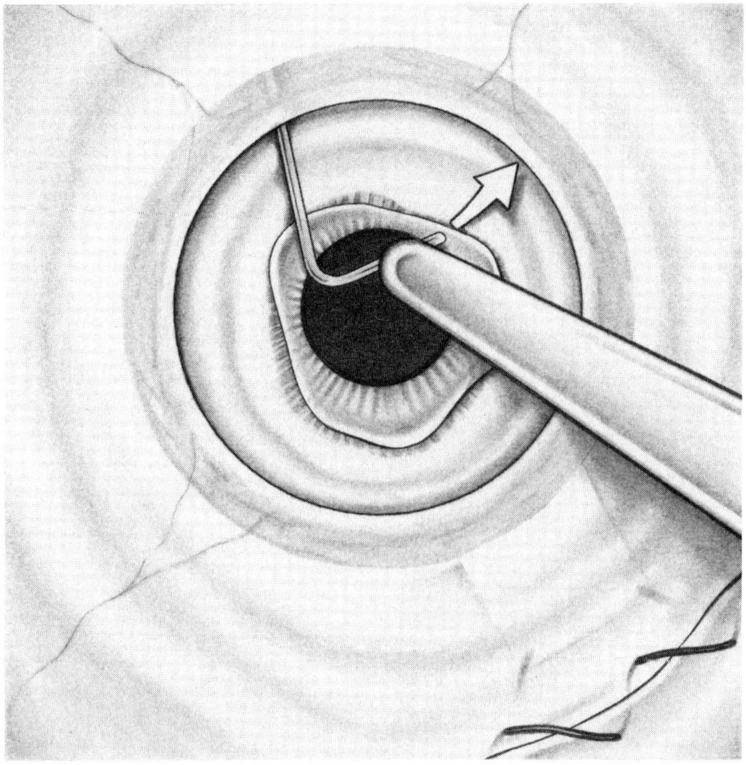

Figure 15–4

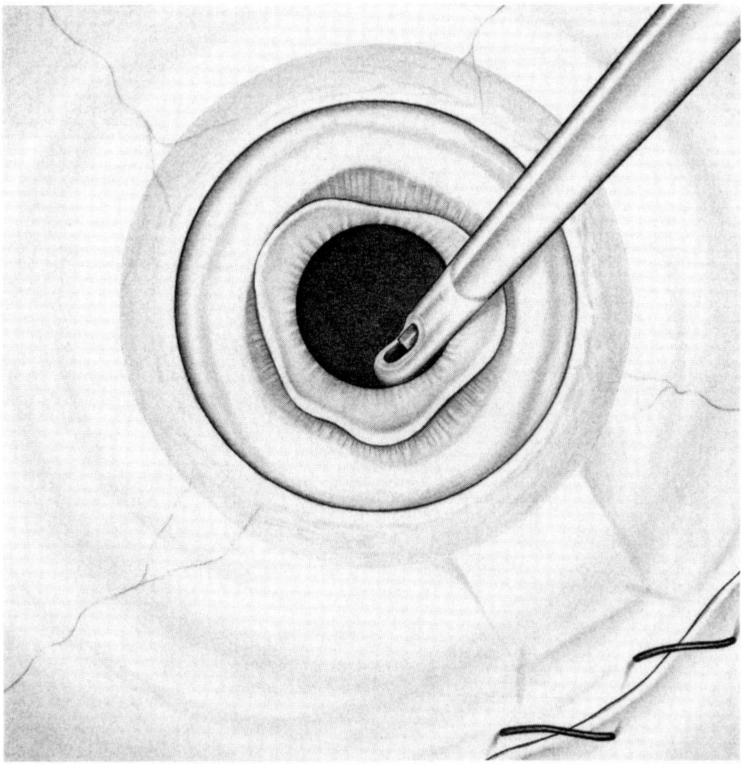

Figure 15–5

Figure 15–6. The vitreous has been cleared from the anterior chamber and replaced by a viscoelastic material. An intracameral miotic agent is injected to constrict the pupil if the spincter is reasonably intact. An anterior chamber lens with flexible haptics is being inserted. The inferior haptic has been placed in the angle, and the superior haptic is being deflected so that it, too, will be placed in the angle 180 degrees away from the inferior haptic. This is easily accomplished in this open-sky technique. The use of a viscoelastic material that lubricates the surface of the iris reduces the chance for entrapment of the iris in the angle by the haptic. However, pupil distortion as the IOL is being inserted indicates iris incarceration in the angle. A spatula inserted under, and gently lifting, the optic frees the iris, and the pupil assumes its rounded shape. As an alternative, a thin spatula is introduced into the angle to lift the haptic and free the iris directly.

Figure 15–7. A donor cornea button 0.25 mm larger than the recipient is sutured into place over a bed of viscoelastic material. The viscoelastic agent may need replacement during the surgery. Four cardinal sutures, placed 90 degrees apart, are inserted in an interrupted fashion, and the running suture is then placed. The running suture is left with both needles attached. If the needle being used becomes bent or unusable or detaches from the suture, the surgeon may use the other needle to complete the suturing in the opposite direction. At the end of this operation, the viscoelastic material is left in the anterior chamber, since exchange with saline may cause contact between the graft endothelium and the anterior chamber IOL. Carbonic anhydrase inhibitors and β-blockers can be used in the early postoperative period until the viscoelastic material has disappeared from the anterior chamber.

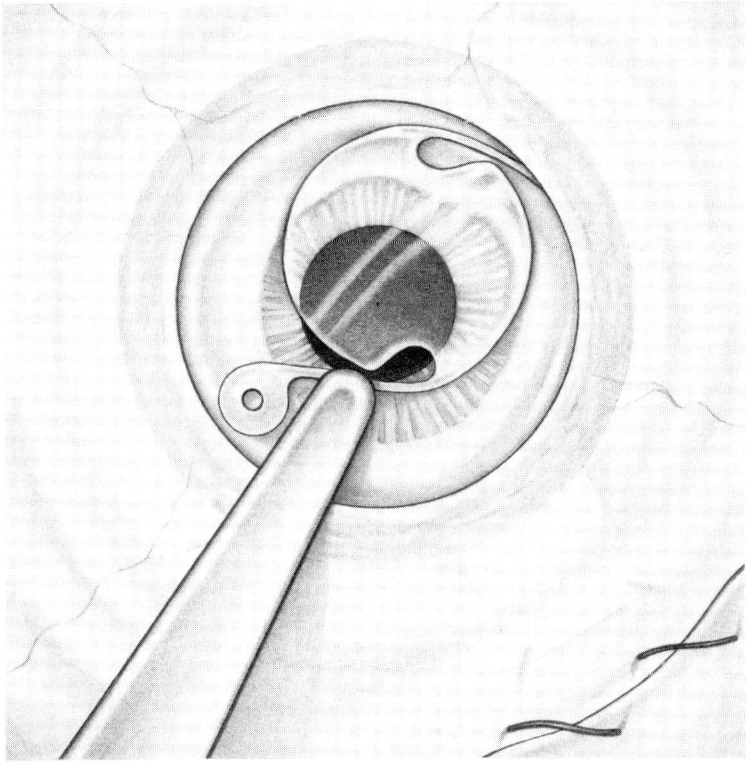

Figure 15–6

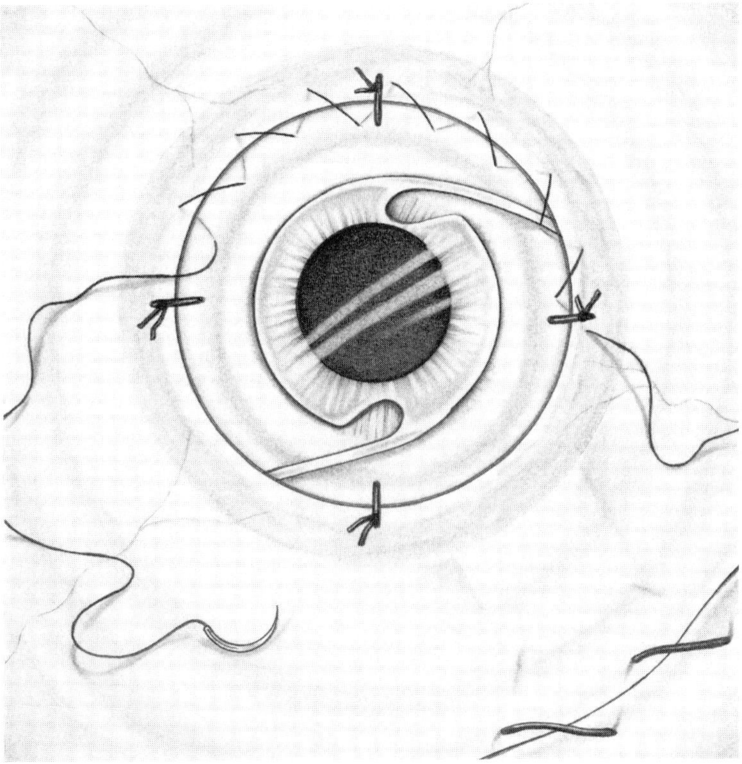

Figure 15–7

Figure 15–8. Cyclodestruction has been accomplished by freezing. A cryoprobe is applied to the region of the ciliary body, and the ice ball is formed. The ice ball should not extend to the clear cornea because the endothelium will be destroyed. The eye has been anesthetized by a retrobulbar block consisting of a mixture of a rapid-onset, shorter-acting and slower-onset, and longer-acting local anesthetic agent.

Figure 15–9. For transscleral YAG cyclodestruction, the eye is totally anesthetized in the manner previously described. A contact YAG delivery system in its free-running thermal mode is aimed at the ciliary epithelium 2–3 mm posterior to the limbus and is retrofocused 3.5 mm into the eye to reach the desired location. Because the total energy of transscleral YAG cyclocoagulation has not been demonstrated, arbitrary levels are used. A typical single session may involve 35 equally spaced applications over the 360 degrees of the ciliary body. The energy level employed varies from 7 to 10 J per site. It has been suggested that the number of applications be titrated against the level of IOP. Whether or not this method is of value is still to be determined. As with the cyclocryo procedure, the YAG transscleral cyclocoagulation may vary in effect from none to phthisis bulbi. This procedure must be used with caution and when alternatives are limited.

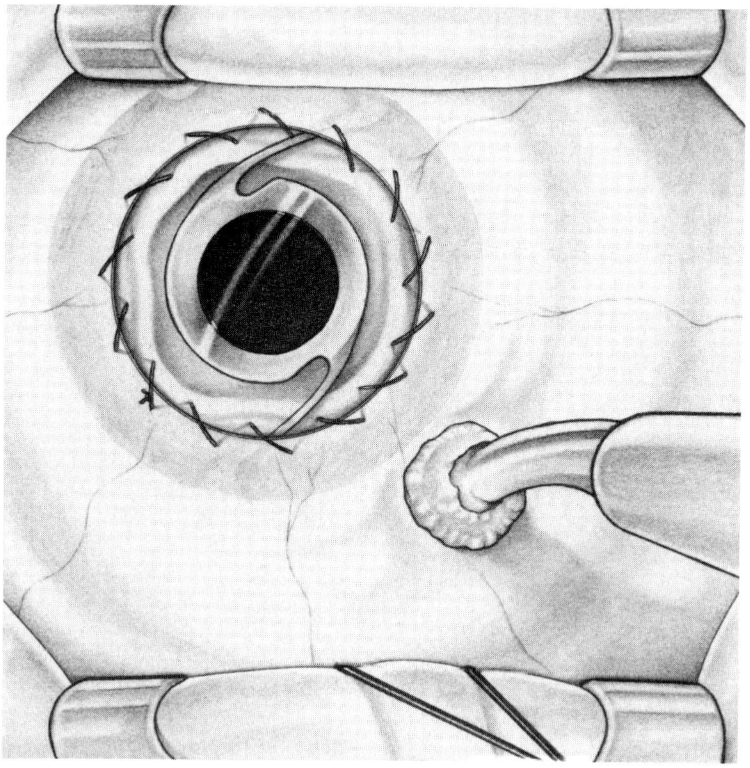

Figure 15–8

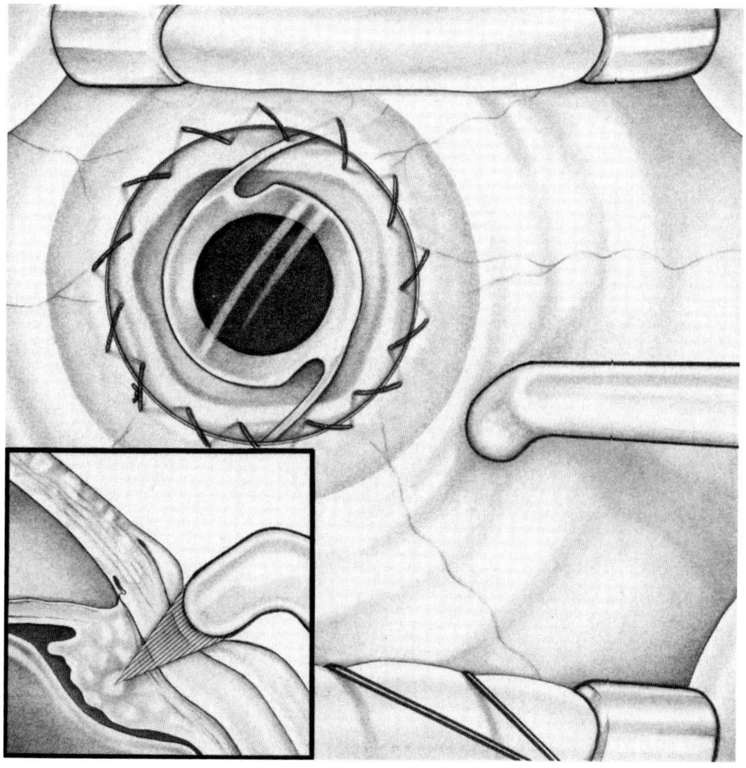

Figure 15–9

Figure 15–10. This cyclodestructive procedure uses focused, high-intensity ultrasound to destroy a portion of the ciliary body. Local anesthesia is required, as previously described. Ultrasound energy not only destroys the ciliary epithelium where aqueous humor is produced but also may thin the sclera, allowing for transscleral filtration. A typical dosage regimen is six applications of 5-seconds duration spaced over the 360 degrees of the ciliary body, with the force zone of the transducer 2.5 mm posterior to the limbus. A force of 3.2 g is applied in a continuous wave. The apparatus must be calibrated daily. It is postulated that most failed filtration blebs fail because of fibrosis within the bleb. It is possible to restore the function of a failed bleb by applying one to two 5-second bursts of ultrasound directly to the bleb. The mechanism of restoration of function is still uncertain, but success has been achieved with this technique.

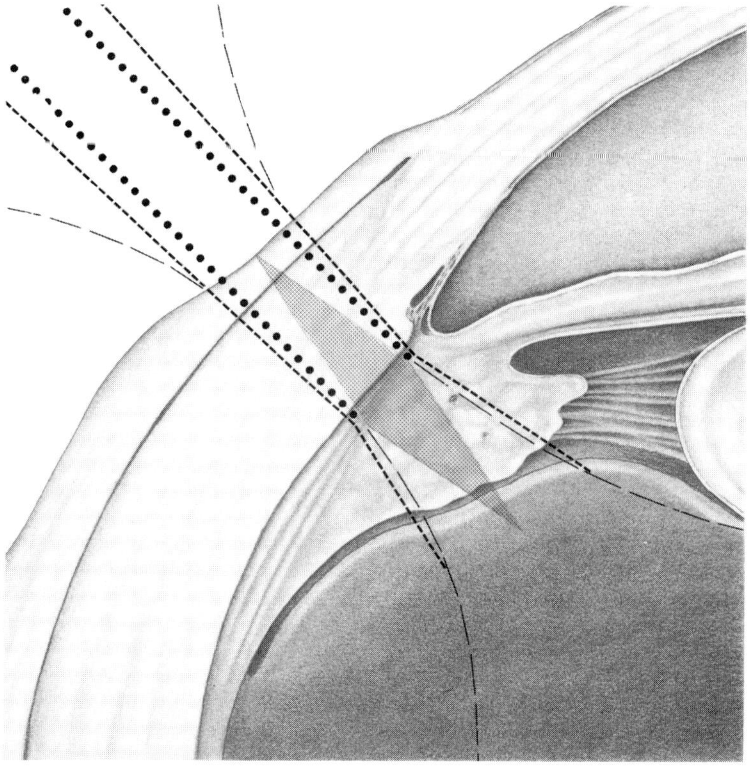

Figure 15–10

Bibliography

Abraham RK, Miller GL. Out-patient argon laser iridectomy for angle-closure glaucoma: A two-year study. *Trans Am Acad Ophthalmol. Otolaryngol* 1975; 79:529.

Ascher KW. Some details of the technique of cyclodialysis. *Am J Ophthalmol.* 1960; 50:1207.

Binkhorst CD, Huber C. Cataract extraction and intraocular lens implantation after fistulizing glaucoma surgery. *Am Intraocular Implant Soc J.* 1981; 7:133.

Boreham CA. Combined extracapsular cataract extraction and posterior chamber intraocular lens implantation and trabeculectomy. *Aust NZ J Ophthalmol.* 1987; 15:201.

Cairns JE. Trabeculectomy. Preliminary report of a new method. *Am J Ophthalmol.* 1968; 5:673.

Chandler PA. Narrow-angle glaucoma. *Arch Ophthalmol.* 1952; 47:695.

Chandler PA, Simmons RJ, Grant WN. Malignant glaucoma. Medical and surgical treatment. *Am J Ophthalmol.* 1968; 66:495.

Coleman DJ, Lizzi FL, Driller J, et al. Therapeutic ultrasound in the treatment of glaucoma. II. Clinical applications. *Ophthalmology.* 1985; 92:347.

Curran EJ. New operation for glaucoma involving a new principle in the etiology and treatment of chronic primary glaucoma. *Arch Ophthalmol.* 1920; 49:131.

Dannheim R. Trabeculotomy. *Trans Am Acad Ophthalmol Otolaryngol.* 1972; 76:375.

Fagadau WR, Obstbaum SA, Herman WK et al. Glaucoma, extracapsular cataract extraction and intraocular lens. In: Abrahamson IA, ed. *Cataract Surgery.* New York: McGraw-Hill; 1986; 126–131.

Handa J, Henry C, Krupin T, et al. Extracapsular cataract extraction with posterior chamber lens implantation in patients with glaucoma. *Arch Ophthalmol.* 1987; 105:765.

Harms H, Dannheim R. Trabeculotomy results and problems. *Adv Ophthalmol.* 1970; 22:121.

Hogan MJ, Alvarado, JA, Weddell JE. *Histology of the Human Eye.* Philadelphia: WB Saunders; 1971.

Kass MA. Cataract extraction in an eye with a filtering bleb. *Ophthalmology.* 1982; 89:871.

Levene R. A new concept of malignant glaucoma. *Arch Ophthalmol.* 1972; 87:497.

Levene R. Triple procedure of extracapsular cataract surgery, posterior chamber lens implantation and glaucoma filter. *J Cataract Refract Surg.* 1986; 12:385.

Lowe RF. Acute angle-closure glaucoma. Acute and subacute attacks. Clinical types. *Trans Ophthalmol Soc Aust.* 1961; 25:65.

Lowe RF. Primary creeping angle-closure glaucoma. *Br J Ophthalmol.* 1964; 48:544.

McGuigan LJB, Gottsch J, Stark WJ, et al. Extracapsular cataract extraction and posterior chamber lens implantation in eyes with pre-existing glaucoma. *Arch Ophthalmol.* 1986; 104:1301.

McPherson SD. Results of external trabeculotomy. *Am J Ophthalmol.* 1973; 75:918.

Obstbaum SA. Glaucoma and intraocular lens implantation. *J Cataract Refract Surg.* 1986; 12:257.

Ohanesian RV, Kim EW. A prospective study of combined extracapsular cataract extraction, posterior chamber lens implantation and trabeculectomy. *Am Intraocular Implant Soc J.* 1985; 1:142.

Oyakawa RT, Maumenee AE. Clear cornea cataract extraction with eyes with functioning filtering blebs. *Am J Ophthalmol.* 1982; 93:294.

Percival SPD. Glaucoma triple procedure of extracapsular cataract extraction, posterior chamber lens implantation and trabeculectomy. *Br J Ophthalmol.* 1985; 69:99.

Pfoff DS. Simultaneous extracapsular cataract extraction, intraocular lens implantation and posterior lip sclerectomy filtering procedure in glaucoma patients. *CLAO J.* 1984; 10:143.

Pollack IP. Chronic angle-closure glaucoma. Diagnosis and treatment in angles of patients that appear open. *Arch Ophthalmol.* 1971; 85:676.

Pollack IP. Use of argon laser energy to produce iridectomies. *Trans Am Ophthalmol Soc.* 1979; 77:674.

Regan EF, Day RM. Cataract extraction after filtering procedures. *Am J Ophthalmol.* 1971; 71:331.

Robin AL, Pollack IP. A comparison of neodymium YAG and argon laser iridectomies. *Ophthalmology.* 1984; 91:1011.

Savage JA, Thomas JV, Belcher CD III, et al. Extracapsular cataract extraction and posterior chamber intraocular lens implantation in glaucomatous eyes. *Ophthalmology.* 1985; 92:1506.

Scheie HG. Retraction of scleral wound edges as a fistulizing procedure for glaucoma. *Am J Ophthalmol.* 1958; 45:220.

Schocket SS, Lakhanpal V, Richards RD. Anterior chamber tube shunt to an encircling band in the treatment of neovascular glaucoma. *Ophthalmology.* 1982; 89:1188.

Schwartz AL, Witten M, Bleiman B, Martin D. Argon laser trabecular surgery in uncontrolled phakic open-angle glaucoma. *Ophthalmology.* 1981; 88:203.

Shaffer RN. *Stereoscopic Manual of Gonioscopy,* St. Louis: CV Mosby; 1962.

Shaffer RN. Prognosis of gonioscopy in primary infantile glaucoma (trabeculodysgenesis). *Trans Am Ophthalmol Soc.* 1982; 80:321.

Shields MB. Trabeculectomy vs full-thickness filtering operation for control of glaucoma. *Ophthalmic Surg.* 1980; 11:498.

Simmons RJ. Malignant glaucoma. *Br J Ophthalmol.* 1972; 56:263.

Simmons RJ, et al. Laser gonioplasty for special problems in angle-closure glaucoma. In: *New Orleans Academy of Ophthalmology; Symposium of Glaucoma.* St. Louis; CV Mosby: 1981.

Simmons RJ, Savage JA, Thomas JV. The glaucomas and extracapsular cataract surgery with posterior chamber lens implantation. In: *New Orleans Academy of Ophthalmology: Symposium of Glaucoma.* St. Louis: CV Mosby; 1985.

Simmons ST, Litoff D, Nichols DA, et al. Extracapsular cataract extraction and posterior chamber lens implantation combined with trabeculectomy in patients with glaucoma. *Am J Ophthalmol.* 1987; 104:465.

Sugar HS. Surgical anatomy for glaucoma. *Surv Ophthalmol.* 1968; 13:143.

Sugar HS. Post-operative cataract in successfully filtering glaucomatous eyes. *Am J Ophthalmol.* 1970; 69:740.

Thomas JV, Simmons RJ, Belcher CD III. Complications of laser trabeculoplasty. *Glaucoma.* 1982; 4:50.

Wand M, Grant WN, Simmons RJ, Hutchinson BT. Plateau iris syndrome. *Trans Am Acad Ophthalmol Otolaryngol.* 1977; 83:122.

Weiss DI, Shaffer RN. Ciliary block (malignant) glaucoma. *Trans Am Acad Ophthalmol Otolaryngol* 1972; 76:450.

Wise, JB, Witter SL. Argon laser therapy for open-angle glaucoma. *Arch Ophthalmol.* 1979; 97:319.

Index

Page numbers in *italics* refer to illustrations